Overview Map Key

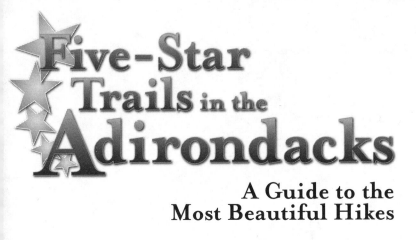

Five-Star Trails in the Adirondacks

A Guide to the Most Beautiful Hikes

Other Books

The Best in Tent Camping: New York State
Canoeing & Kayaking New York
Easy Hikes Close to Home: New York City
Peaceful Places: New York City
60 Hikes within 60 Miles: New York City

Five-Star Trails in the Adirondacks

A Guide to the Most Beautiful Hikes

TIM STARMER

MENASHA RIDGE PRESS

Cover design by Scott McGrew
Text by Ian Szymkowiak/Palace Press International
All photographs by Tim Starmer
Cartography and elevation profiles by Scott McGrew
Indexing by Jan Mucciarone
Cover photos: Crane Mountain (Hike 21)
Frontispiece: Fire tower at Owls Head Mountain (Hike 32)

Library of Congress Cataloging-in-Publication Data

    Starmer, Timothy, 1975-
       Five-star trails in the Adirondacks : a guide to the most beautiful
       hikes / Tim Starmer. — 1st ed.
          p. cm.
       Includes index.
       ISBN-13: 978-0-89732-683-4
       ISBN-10: 0-89732-683-0
    1. Hiking—New York (State)—Adirondack Mountains—Guidebooks.
    2. Trails—New York (State)—Adirondack Mountains—Guidebooks.
    3. Adirondack Mountains (N.Y.)—Guidebooks. I. Title.
      GV199.42.N652A34735 2010
      917.47'53--dc22

                    2010020130

Menasha Ridge Press
P.O. Box 43673
Birmingham, Alabama 35243
www.menasharidge.com

DISCLAIMER
This book is meant only as a guide to select trails in the vicinity of the Adirondacks and does not guarantee your safety in any way—you hike at your own risk. Neither Menasha Ridge Press nor Tim Starmer is liable for property loss or damage, personal injury, or death that may result from accessing or hiking the trails described in the following pages. Please be aware that hikers have been injured in the Adirondacks. Be especially cautious when walking on or near boulders, steep inclines, and drop-offs, and do not attempt to explore terrain that may be beyond your abilities. To help ensure an uneventful hike, please read carefully the introduction to this book, and perhaps get further safety information and guidance from other sources. Familiarize yourself thoroughly with the areas you intend to visit before venturing out. Ask questions and prepare for the unforeseen. Familiarize yourself with current weather reports, maps of the area you intend to visit, and any relevant area regulations.

Table of Contents

Dedication

This book is dedicated to my parents, who first inspired in me a love of the great outdoors and helped in innumerable ways in completing this book.

Acknowledgments

FIRST AND FOREMOST, I WOULD LIKE TO THANK EVERYONE who braved the trails with me and endured my repetitious mumblings into my voice recorder. Your company was appreciated and helpful.

Second, I must acknowledge all the work that my parents contributed to this project, from editing my rough drafts to retyping hikes I lost when my computer crashed to loaning me a car when my truck broke down, sadly more than once.

Finally, I would like to acknowledge the tireless efforts of all the trail crews who maintain the thousands of miles of trails in the Adirondacks. Your work is greatly admired and appreciated.

Preface

WORKING ON THIS BOOK WAS DEFINITELY AN EXPERIENCE to remember. I lost two hard drives; had to rewrite a handful of hikes from memory; fried a camera, a voice recorder, and a GPS unit; sprained my ankle; was nearly blown off a mountaintop; and was stranded in the middle of the Adirondacks when my truck broke down and AAA redefined 24/7 service as weekdays only during business hours. It was memorable and—quite simply—great. Planning and replanning hikes, followed by days in the woods, is more than most hikers can ask for; to do so in the Adirondacks is definitely more than most get.

For those who don't know, the Adirondack Park is huge. The park's boundaries encompass 9,375 square miles, which is larger than each of the states of Rhode Island, Delaware, Connecticut, New Jersey, and New Hampshire. It is only 240 square miles smaller than Vermont. Compared to national parks, the Adirondack Park is larger than Grand Canyon, Yellowstone, Yosemite, Great Smoky Mountains, and Big Bend national parks combined. In fact its boundaries, also known as the blue line, encompass more acreage than any of the national parks in the lower 48 states. Not all of the land within the blue line is owned or managed by the state. Towns, villages, and two entire counties, as well as vast tracts of privately held land, lie within its boundaries. However, don't let the land classification fool you— the park is truly a vast wilderness. Of the 6.1 million acres, 45%, or 2.7 million acres, is owned by the state, though donations and purchases continue to expand the state-owned land. Of the remaining land, less than 1% is municipal property and about 6% is classified as low-level residential, which is almost equivalent to the amount of acreage of water within the park. The remaining land is either rural or privately owned forests.

No matter how you frame it, the park is a huge wilderness, and you sense it almost immediately after passing the blue line. As you drive toward any of the hundreds of trailheads, you can feel the forest encroaching on the fields and houses along the roads. You know that the boundary between civilization and a sprawling wilderness is just beyond the tree line. Soon the forests have overrun manicured lawns, and fields give way to staggering boulders and craggy cliffs that loom close to the roadside. You sense that at any point, you could stop your car, step out into the woods, and within feet completely leave civilization behind. All the while, should you choose to stop at a diner for lunch in between hikes, forget camera batteries, need to refuel, or need replacement gear, there is typically a spot to resupply within a half hour of a trailhead. This is the charm of the Adirondacks: Vast wilderness, in which you can spend days in solitude, is at your fingertips, and yet civilization is still close at hand. For many beginning hikers this is a great comfort, while experienced hikers can revel in the idea of a warm meal or cold drink at the end of a journey.

My goal in writing this book was to cater to both beginning and experienced hikers, to provide easy and challenging hikes in all corners of the park. I could have easily found 40 hikes in any single region, and all would have been rewarding. Some of the hikes will be familiar, others less known, but all are rewarding examples of the many facets of the Adirondack Park and its thousands of miles of trails.

Recommended Hikes

Hikes by Category

Introduction

About This Book

AN ESTIMATED 6 MILLION TO 10 MILLION tourists visit Adirondack Park every year. With 3,000 lakes, 30,000 miles of rivers and streams, 2,000 miles of hiking trails, and more than 100 mountains, it is no surprise. Unique is barely adequate to describe the character of the Adirondacks. It stands out as the largest park in the lower 48 states; however, unlike its rivals, it's managed solely by the state. It has the only mountains in the Northeast that are not geologically Appalachian. The mountains, though geologically new, are from old rock. Ecologically, the park lies on the transition of the boreal forests of the north and deciduous hardwood forests of the south. The Adirondack region was also at the forefront of conservation when, in 1894, the Forever Wild character of the Forest Preserve was added to the state constitution, making it the only preserve with constitutional protection.

New mountains from old rock seem a contradiction, but this is what makes the Adirondack Mountains distinct from their Appalachian neighbors along the East Coast. Unlike the Appalachian Mountains, which were formed by plate tectonics, the Adirondack Mountains were formed by uplift. Imagine an iceberg with enough weight on it to keep it beneath the water's surface. Remove the weight, and the iceberg surges above the surface. A similar process exists today in the Adirondacks. Indeed, the Adirondacks are still rising. Granted, the rate is only about 3 millimeters per year, but this rate is faster than the rate of erosion, so the mountains are creeping ever upward. So the next time someone comments that life was tougher in his day, you can quip that at least his mountains were shorter. The protruding old rock was formed when the Adirondacks were part of a giant inland sea. Over millennia, miles of sediment were deposited and later transformed by high pressure and heat into metamorphosed rock. The deposits and formation took place 1 billion years ago, and the metamorphosed rock lay miles beneath the surface until erosion removed enough material for a 160-mile-wide bulge to begin swelling above the surrounding landscape about 5 million years ago. Further stages of uplift, erosion, and the scouring of the landscape by great ice sheets have exposed the meta-morphosed rock and caused the uplift to increase. These powerful forces of uplift, erosion, and scouring transformed the region into the rugged wilderness we see today.

Native Americans did not settle in the Adirondacks but rather used them mostly as hunting grounds. As Europeans began to explore and settle the continent, they stayed on the fringes of the wilderness, mostly along the shores of Lake George and Lake Champlain. These lakes formed a major strategic territory for mastery of the continent. The Iroquois and Algonquin often fought over the water route long before the pitched battles of the French and Indian War. During this war, the French controlled Fort Carillon, later named Fort Ticonderoga, on the northern shore of Lake George, while the English controlled Fort William Henry on the south end. James Fenimore Cooper's novel *Last of the Mohicans* depicts one of the major events in this contest over the water route: the surrender of Fort William Henry followed by a massacre of the retreating English troops on their way to Fort Edward. The magnitude of the massacre has been estimated from dozens to thousands, though it is generally agreed that Cooper's depiction is exaggerated. Later epic battles were fought during this war and then again during the American Revolution. However, during all this time, the interior of the Adirondack wilderness was rarely broached.

Settlement in the region did not begin in earnest until the 1800s, when the Industrial Revolution's growing demand for natural resources turned its eyes on the vast stands of timber and newly discovered veins of iron ore. Great wealth was created during the Gilded Age, and consequently, the Adirondacks became a popular vacation area with great camps and resorts. At the same time, conservation and a love of the outdoors were taking hold of the public, and the devastation of the Adirondack forests became a growing concern among these newly arrived vacationers. In 1885 the state created the Adirondack Forest Preserve, which directed that "the lands now or hereafter constituting the Forest Preserve be forever kept as wild forest lands." Later in 1892 the state established the Adirondack State Park and drew the infamous blue line to encompass the Adirondack Forest Preserve, as well as millions of acres of private land. Despite these protections, the forest preserve law was still violated; in 1894 the "forever wild" clause was added to the state constitution of New York. Tourism continued to thrive in the region and saw increases after World War I and World War II. Second homes within the park became a growing concern, and in 1971 the Adirondack Park Agency was created to develop and oversee land-use plans with consideration of the forever wild clause.

Today the park still maintains a delicate balance between the interests of private landholders and the public lands owned by the state. To say that tourism is a mainstay of the region is an understatement. There are 130,000 people living year-round in the 9,375 square miles encompassed by the blue line, with an estimated 200,000 seasonal residents and anywhere from 6 million to 10 million tourists. So odds are that if you ask someone for directions, the person won't be from around there. Tourism is year-round, with winter attracting snowmobilers, skiers, and snowshoers in as many numbers as summer's vacationers and fall's hunters. About the only downtime is in early spring during the mud season.

The hikes within this book are meant to provide a wide range of experiences over the vast area of the park. For decades the park has informally been divided into regions in various ways. The Department of Environmental Conservation (DEC) has regions that sprawl across the blue line; counties divide the park but also cross the line; and varying tourist centers divide the region based on proximity to major lakes or towns.

Most people adhere to the six regions devised by the Adirondack Mountain Club (ADK) in their series of Forest Preserve guidebooks. I have similarly divided the region because it proves useful for hikers seeking nearby trails or additional maps and is generally understood by most hikers as the way the park is divided. Though regions often overlap, some distinctions between the regions help to describe the area to be explored.

WEST-CENTRAL REGION

Along the western border of the park are the foothills that lead to the Adirondack Mountains. Few mountains are in this area; most trails follow the shores of lakes and rivers and feature generally flat terrain. The few mountain trails in this area are well liked, so expect lots of company. Indeed the region, especially around the towns of Old Forge and Inlet, is extremely popular with tourists. Many of the great camps were built here, and it serves as a staging point for longer expeditions into the Adirondacks. Several excellent campgrounds, outdoors stores, and outfitters are in the area, making it a good point to resupply or pick up forgotten items as you head deeper into the park. It does not take long to leave the vestiges of civilization behind here, so the purist should not shun this region simply because it is well known.

CENTRAL REGION

As might be expected, the Central Region lies in the center of many of the other Adirondack regions; consequently many of its trailheads lie literally across the street from a trail in another region. Many of the trails described in this region are unmarked and considered bushwhacks but generally are well trodden. Additionally, these trails follow the course of streams, so navigating them should be relatively easy. The area is essentially bound by NY 28 to the north and NY 8 to the south. Several mountains are in this region, though most are easy to climb. An abundance of waterfalls in this region makes it an excellent area for exploring waterscapes. Many of the campgrounds in the area provide solitude and scenery, making them excellent staging areas for exploring all the regions in the park.

EASTERN REGION

Hikes in this region focus on the shores of Lake George and feature spectacular vistas from the mountains that surround the beautiful lake. The southern tip of Lake George is full of tourist trappings and won't be high on the list for most devoted hikers. However, it does provide a good staging area, the opportunity to reconnect with civilization, and quick access to the excellent wilderness areas nearby. Pharaoh Lake and Mountain are featured in the book but cover just a small portion of the vast Pharaoh Lake Wilderness Area.

SOUTHERN REGION

The southern foothills are not known for their mountains, so it may seem odd that the two mountains featured here are actually some of the steepest hikes. They are not as tall as those in the High Peaks, but their straight-up ascents make them reasonably challenging yet well within the novice hiker's range. Similar to the West-Central and Central regions, the terrain here is mostly level, and lakes and other bodies of water are the primary focus of trails. Several unmarked trails are also featured in this region but are easy to follow with a little navigational experience.

NORTHERN REGION

The Northern Region looks and feels like a giant river basin. The mostly level terrain is dotted with innumerable ponds, lakes, and marshes, which are all bisected by a network of streams and winding rivers. Floodwood Loop and High Falls Loop described in this guide typify the region and are fascinating areas to explore. Not as built-up or commercial as other areas in the park, the Northern Region is definitely the most remote and probably the hardest area to resupply in. Cranberry Lake, Tupper Lake, and Saranac are the largest developed areas, but you'll pass through them quickly. Hikes here are generally more secluded; however, as is the case in most regions, the peaks attract the most hikers.

High Peaks Region

Rugged and wild, the High Peaks typify the Adirondacks. Hikers who put off venturing into the High Peaks Region for decades often never return to their earlier stomping grounds once they get a taste of the High Peaks. Generally trails here are steeper, cliffs and waterfalls are taller, and the sheer quantity of peaks in this region changes your view of what rugged looks and feels like. This book offers just a sampling of the adventures that lie in the High Peaks and leans toward the beginner level for the region. However, beginner High Peaks trails are typically more difficult than more advanced trails in other regions.

How to Use This Guidebook
The Overview Map and Key

Use the overview map on the inside front cover to assess the exact location of each hike's primary trailhead. Each hike's number appears on the overview map, on the map key facing the overview map, and in the table of contents. A hike's full profile is easy to locate as you flip through the book—just watch for the hike number at the top of each page.

The book is organized by region, as indicated in the table of contents, and the hikes within each region are noted as day hikes or overnight hikes. They are also labeled as out-and-back, loop, or point-to-point routes in the table of contents. A map legend that details the symbols found on trail maps appears on the inside back cover.

TRAIL MAPS

Each hike contains a detailed map that shows the trailhead, the route, significant features, facilities, and landmarks such as creeks, overlooks, and peaks. I gathered map data by carrying a GPS unit (Garmin eTrex) while hiking. This data was downloaded into a digital mapping program (TOPO USA) and then processed by expert cartographers to produce the highly accurate maps found in this book. Each trailhead's GPS coordinates are included with each profile (see below).

ELEVATION PROFILES

Each hike description is accompanied by a detailed elevation profile that corresponds directly to the trail map. The elevation profile enables you to easily visualize how the trail rises and falls. Key points along the way are labeled. Note the number of feet between each tick mark on the vertical axis (the height scale). To avoid making flat hikes look steep and steep hikes appear flat, height scales are used throughout the book to provide an accurate assessment of each hike's climbing difficulty.

GPS TRAILHEAD COORDINATES

This book also includes the GPS coordinates for each trailhead in two formats: latitude and longitude and Universal Transverse Mercator (UTM). Latitude and longitude coordinates tell you where you are by locating a point west (latitude) of the zero-degree meridian line that passes through Greenwich, England, and north or south of the zero-degree (longitude) line, the equator, that belts the Earth.

Topographic maps show latitude and longitude in addition to UTM grid lines. Known as UTM coordinates, the numbers index a specific point using a grid method. The survey datum used to arrive at the coordinates in this book is WGS 84 (versus NAD 27 or WGS 83). For readers who own a GPS unit, whether handheld or onboard a vehicle, the latitude and longitude or UTM coordinates provided on the last page of each hike may be entered into the GPS unit. Just make sure that your GPS unit is set to navigate using WGS84 datum. Now you can navigate directly to the trailhead.

Most trailheads begin in parking areas, but some trailheads are a short walk from a parking area. In those cases, a handheld unit is necessary to continue the GPS navigation process. That said, readers can easily access all trailheads in this book by using the directions given, the overview map, and the trail map, which shows at least one major road leading into the area. But for those who enjoy using the latest GPS technology to navigate, the necessary data has been provided. A brief explanation of the UTM coordinates for Giant's Nubble (page 250) follows.

UTM Zone (WGS 84): 18T
Easting: 0598595.1
Northing: 4889319.9

The UTM zone number (18) refers to one of the 60 vertical zones of the UTM projection. Each zone is 6 degrees wide. The UTM zone letter (T) refers to one of the 20 horizontal zones that span from 80 degrees south to 84 degrees north. The easting number (0598595.1) indicates in meters how far east or west a point is from the central meridian of the zone. Increasing easting coordinates indicate that you are moving east; decreasing easting coordinates indicate that you are moving west. The northing number (4889319.9) shows in meters how far you are from the equator. Above and below the equator, increasing northing coordinates indicate that you are traveling north; decreasing northing coordinates indicate that you are traveling south. To enhance your outdoor experiences with GPS technology, refer to *GPS Outdoors: A Practical Guide For Outdoor Enthusiasts* (Menasha Ridge Press).

THE HIKE PROFILE

In addition to a map, each hike contains a concise but informative narrative of the hike from beginning to end. This descriptive text is enhanced with at-a-glance ratings and information, GPS-based trail-head coordinates, and accurate driving directions leading you from a major road to the parking area most convenient to the trailhead.

At the beginning of each hike, a box gives hikers quick access to pertinent information: the quality of scenery, the condition of the trail, the hike's appropriateness for children, the difficulty of the hike, the degree of solitude expected, hike distance, approximate hiking time, and outstanding highlights of the trip. The first five categories are rated using a five-star system. Below is an example.

37 Giant's **Nubble**

SCENERY: ✪ ✪ ✪ ✪ ✪	DISTANCE: *4.4 miles*
TRAIL CONDITION: ✪ ✪ ✪ ✪	HIKING TIME: *3–4 hours*
CHILDREN: ✪ ✪	OUTSTANDING FEATURES: *Spectacular*
DIFFICULTY: ✪ ✪ ✪ ✪	*waterfall, primitive campsites, outstanding views*
SOLITUDE: ✪ ✪ ✪	

In this example, five stars indicate that the scenery is very picturesque with excellent views and/or unique features (three stars would be a typical hike in the woods with some added scenic interest). The trail condition is very good (one star would mean the trail is muddy, rocky, overgrown, or otherwise compromised). The two-star rating for children denotes that children who are experienced and enjoy long hikes would be appropriate (one star would mean that only the most gung-ho and physically fit children should go). Four stars for difficulty indicate that it is a relatively tough hike (five stars would indicate that it's strenuous). Three stars for solitude mean that you can expect to encounter people on the trail but mostly in passing (you may well be elbowing your way up the trail on one-star hikes).

Distances given are absolute, but hiking times are based on an average hiking speed of 2 to 3 miles per hour, with time built in for pauses at overlooks and brief rests.

Following this summary information is a brief description of the hike. A more detailed account follows, in which trail junctions, stream crossings, and trailside features are noted, along with their distance from the trailhead. Flip through the book, read the brief descriptions, and choose the hikes that appeal to you. A list of recommended hikes (see pages xiv–xvi) also helps you choose a hike to fit your mood and group.

Weather

WEATHER IN THE ADIRONDACKS SHOULD NOT BE TAKEN LIGHTLY. Conditions can change rapidly during all seasons, and the conditions at the base of a tall mountain will certainly not be the same at the top. When I set out to hike Ampersand Mountain, it was a bright, sunny day in the height of summer. Clouds rolled in, and an unpredicted and severe thunderstorm set in quickly with little warning. Those at the peak sheltered near large boulders at the top, while those at the base turned back. Unfortunately, I was caught in the tree line just below the peak. The situation soon became precarious, as the wind howled and bent trees near the point of snapping. Heavy rains flooded the path, making footing slick. Turning around meant passing through an area where blowdown was likely and unpredictable, and the steep, rocky path became slicker by the minute—hurrying would not be an option. I managed to shelter near the top, where the tree line broke, and descended during a brief break in the weather. When I finally reached my truck, the system had passed, clear skies prevailed, and little evidence of the severe storm remained. Despite raingear, my clothes told a different story than the skies. So as a rule, prepare for the worst case, even if the best is forecasted.

Generally speaking, the Adirondacks are cooler than the rest of New York. This is a welcome respite during summer, but it also means that snow may fall from September into May. Summer temperatures rarely go into the 90s, while winter temperatures often go below zero. Average temperatures are in the mild range, with high 70s typical in summer. Though it varies year to year, the hiking season is generally between May and October, though proper attire and preparation is always advised.

Snowshoeing and skiing are also popular in this area, and all of the trails described in this book can be done with snowshoes. Indeed, though temperatures often plummet below zero, snowshoeing is often the best way to get some solitude on the more popular trails. Late March and early April, also called the mud season, are likely the least advisable times for hiking the Adirondacks, and most seasonal roads are closed during this time. Additionally, trail erosion is worst during mud season, and the DEC has asked that hikers refrain from hiking in areas above 3,000 feet, as the erosion is particularly damaging to alpine vegetation at this time.

Water

WITH COOL TEMPERATURES, 3,000 LAKES AND PONDS, as well as 30,000 miles of streams and rivers, concern for water may seem overly cautious. However *Giardia lamblia,* commonly referred to as giardia, has contaminated many water sources in the Adirondacks. Also known as "beaver fever," the intestinal parasite causes, well, put politely, intestinal problems, weeks after ingestion, the likes of which most would not wish on their enemies. The words watery, explosive, foul, and rotten have also been used to describe the aftereffects, so caution is simply necessary. The single-celled organism is transported by all warm-blooded animals, which in turn contaminate water sources. Because beavers are typically in the water and fail to wash their hands, or even leave the water, after using the lavatory, they are often the culprits of the spread and have been rewarded with the disease's moniker. Beavers also abound in the Adirondacks, and many, if not most, streams have beaver activity in or around them. Humans are also culprits in the transporting and contamination of water sources. To prevent contamination, follow the appropriate guidelines for waste disposal as outlined by the DEC and as described later in this book (see page 23).

Aside from the inherent risks of drinking untreated water, many of the ponds and lakes are fairly stagnant and taste bad. Effective and proper water treatment is essential for using any source found along the trail. Boiling water for 2 to 3 minutes is always a safe measure, as are iodine tablets, approved chemical mixes, filtration units rated for giardia, and UV filtration. Some of these methods (such as filtration with an added carbon filter) remove bad tastes, while others add their own taste. My suggestion is to research a filtration method, devise a way to make it palatable, always carry along a means to purify water, and carry enough water for the hike. A cool drink waiting in the car is always a welcome reward, but it's of little use on the trail. Carry a means of purification to help in a pinch or if you underestimate your consumption, but always bring a couple of water bottles for everyone in your group.

How much is enough? Well, one simple physiological fact should convince you to err on the side of excess when deciding how much water to pack: A hiker working hard in 90°F heat needs approximately 10 quarts of fluid per day. That's 2.5 gallons—12 large water bottles or 16 small ones. In other words, pack along one or two bottles even for short hikes. Hydrate prior to your hike, carry (and drink) six ounces of water for every mile you plan to hike, and hydrate after the hike.

 # Clothing

Proper attire will make the difference between enjoying the trail and having a miserable experience. In the worst case it could even save your life. I add these words of caution not to be dramatic but because it is so easy to disregard simple considerations, especially on short trips and especially when it comes to clothing. Weather is unpredictable; trail conditions change or become impassable; we overestimate our abilities and underestimate required hiking times; and wrong turns happen. On a backpacking trip we are usually prepared for these eventualities because we know that we will be out in the woods for a long time. Don't get me wrong—I'm not advocating hiring a Sherpa or bringing your entire wardrobe, but proper attire at the outset will mitigate most problems.

A few simple guidelines will avert most inconveniences and help you avoid most disasters. When hiking, wear hiking boots and not sandals, flip-flops, or sneakers. Trails in the Adirondacks are hardened, which means they traverse rocky paths to minimize erosion. It protects the forest but is hard on the ankles, so wear proper footwear. Proper layering is also essential to comfortable hiking without excessive perspiration, so wear or pack all layers for the season. Dress for the day and prepare for the worst. This means that if it is 75°F and sunny, dress in what is comfortable for you, but bring raingear and do not leave it in the car if the weather looks good. In spring or fall always wear or bring a wool hat and gloves. On the trail I wear pants with zip-off legs and always bring a pack with food and water, as well as a change of socks and shirt, raingear, gaiters, and a warm hat. With these few extra items, you are prepared for any condition or eventuality without adding much weight. In fall, winter, and spring, remember that "cotton kills," so wear silk, wool, or synthetics. In summer cotton may be passable but *only* if you bring a change of clothing that will not get wet. In an emergency you are only prepared with what you have on or with you. Remember, the worst may include spending the night in the woods in spring or fall when daytime and nighttime temperatures vary drastically, so be prepared.

Essential Gear

ALONG WITH PROPER ATTIRE, THERE ARE SEVERAL OTHER essential items that every hiker should bring with him or her, even on short day hikes. As I alluded to in the section about clothing, no one plans on a one-hour hike turning into a night lost in the woods, but it happens all the time to novice and experienced hikers alike. A complete list of items to bring along for day trips and backpacking trips is found in Appendix B (see page 276), but I've listed the essentials here. These items can be carried in your pockets if carefully packed, but carrying a light backpack is often easier. In addition to carrying the items listed below, you need to know how to use them, especially the ones involving navigation.

WATER: Bring a means to carry it and purify it (for example, water bottle and iodine or a filter)

NAVIGATION: Always carry a map, preferably a topo and a trail map with route description, and high-quality compass

KNIFE OR MULTITOOL: A pocket knife and/or multitool with pliers

LIGHT: A flashlight or headlamp with extra bulb and batteries

FIRE: Windproof matches and/or a lighter, as well as a fire starter

FIRST-AID KIT: See below for a list of basic items to be kept in your kit

EXTRA FOOD: Trail mix, granola bars, or other high-energy foods

EXTRA CLOTHES: Raingear, warm hat, gloves, change of socks and shirt

SUN PROTECTION: sunglasses, lip balm, sunblock, and a sun hat

First-aid Kit

A TYPICAL FIRST-AID KIT MAY CONTAIN MORE ITEMS THAN YOU MIGHT THINK NECESSARY. These are just the basics. Prepackaged kits in waterproof bags (Atwater Carey and Adventure Medical make a variety of kits) are available. Even though quite a few items are listed here, they pack down into a small space.

Ace bandages or Spenco joint wraps

Adhesive bandages

Antibiotic ointment
(*Neosporin or the generic equivalent*)

Athletic tape

Benadryl or the generic equivalent,
diphenhydramine (*in case of allergic
reactions*)

Blister kit (*such as Moleskin or
Spenco Second Skin*)

Butterfly-closure bandages

Epinephrine in a prefilled syringe
(*for people known to have severe allergic
reactions to such things as bee stings, usually by
prescription only*)

Gauze and compress pads (*one roll and a
half dozen 4- by 4-inch pads*)

Hydrogen peroxide or iodine

Ibuprofen or acetaminophen

Insect repellent

Matches or a pocket lighter

Sunscreen

Tweezers

Whistle (*more effective at signaling rescuers
than your voice*)

General Safety

TO SOME POTENTIAL MOUNTAIN ENTHUSIASTS, the deep
woods seem inordinately dark and perilous. It is the fear of the
unknown that causes this anxiety. No doubt, potentially dangerous situations can occur outdoors, but as long as you use sound
judgment and prepare yourself before hitting the trail, you'll be
much safer in the woods than in most urban areas of the country.
It is better to look at a backcountry hike as a fascinating chance to
discover the unknown rather than a chance for potential disaster.
If you're new to the game, I'd suggest starting out easy and finding
a person who knows more to help you out. In addition, here are a
few tips to make your trip safer and easier.

- ALWAYS LET SOMEONE KNOW YOUR PLANS IN ADVANCE.
  Tell your safety person which trails you will be on, when and where
  you expect to depart from, and when and where you expect to return.
  Although you are primarily responsible for your safety, your safety person is your backup plan and will alert rescuers where to look for you.

Remember to tell your safety person all changes in your plans and check in to let them know your trip went well.

· **ALWAYS SIGN IN AND OUT OF THE TRAIL REGISTERS PROVIDED.** If you are hiking several trails, it will alert rescuers where you are and, sometimes more important, where you are not.

While getting lost is unlikely on shorter trails, injury is a distinct possibility, as indicated by numerous warning signs of precipitous cliffs. While bravado may foolishly deter people from using the registers for the first reason, the second reason may appeal more to their self-interest. Additionally the DEC and the state base many of their trail-maintenance and funding decisions on trail registers. If you want to see your favorite trails maintained or want more like them, then let the registers act as your democratic voice in the wilderness.

· **NEVER RELY ON A CELL PHONE, BUT BRING ONE JUST IN CASE.** Reception is spotty at best and virtually nonexistent in most areas—and your phone won't work as kindling.

· **ALWAYS CARRY FOOD AND WATER,** whether you are planning to go overnight or not. Food will give you energy, help keep you warm, and sustain you in an emergency until help arrives. You never know if a stream will be nearby when you become thirsty. Bring potable water or treat water before drinking it from a stream. Boil or filter all found water before drinking it.

· **STAY ON DESIGNATED TRAILS.** Most hikers get lost when they leave the path. Even on the most clearly marked trails, there is usually a point where you have to stop and consider what direction to head. If you become disoriented, don't panic. As soon as you think that you may be off track, stop, assess your current direction, and then retrace your steps to the point where you went astray. Using a map, a compass, and this book, and keeping in mind what you have passed thus far, reorient yourself and trust your judgment on which way to continue. If you become absolutely unsure of how to continue, return to your vehicle the way you came in. Should you become completely lost and have no idea how to return to the trailhead, remaining in place along the trail and waiting for help is most often the best option for adults and always the best option for children.

- **BE ESPECIALLY CAREFUL WHEN CROSSING STREAMS.** Whether you are fording the stream or crossing on a log, make every step count. If you have any doubt about maintaining your balance on a log, ford the stream instead. When crossing, use a trekking pole or stout stick for balance and face upstream as you cross. If a stream seems too deep to ford, turn back. Whatever is on the other side is not worth risking your life.

- **BE CAREFUL AT OVERLOOKS.** While these areas may provide spectacular views, they are potentially hazardous. Stay back from the edge of outcrops and be absolutely sure of your footing; a misstep can mean a nasty and possibly fatal fall.

- **STANDING DEAD TREES AND STORM-DAMAGED LIVING TREES** pose a real hazard to hikers and tent campers. These trees may have loose or broken limbs that could fall at any time. When choosing a spot to rest or a backcountry campsite, look up.

- **KNOW THE SYMPTOMS OF HYPOTHERMIA.** Shivering and forgetfulness are the two most common indicators of this stealthy killer. Hypothermia can occur at any elevation, even in the summer, especially when the hiker is wearing lightweight cotton clothing. If symptoms arise, get the victim shelter, hot liquids, and dry clothes or a dry sleeping bag.

- **TAKE ALONG YOUR BRAIN.** A cool, calculating mind is the single most important asset on the trail. Think before you act. Watch your step. Plan ahead. Avoiding accidents is the best way to ensure a rewarding and relaxing hike.

- **ASK QUESTIONS.** State forest and park employees are there to help. It's a lot easier to ask advice beforehand, and it will help you avoid a mishap away from civilization when it's too late to amend an error.

Animal, Insect, and Plant Hazards

Black Bears

BLACK BEARS ARE FOUND THROUGHOUT NEW YORK STATE but are most frequently encountered in the Adirondacks and occasionally in the Catskills. Though attacks by black bears are virtually unheard of, a bear tearing up your gear or rummaging about outside your tent will give anyone a start. If you encounter a bear at your campsite or while hiking, remain calm and never run away. Make loud noises to scare off the bear and back away slowly.

Black bears normally avoid humans, but you should always leave them an escape route if you encounter them. They can sprint up to 35 mph and are strong swimmers and great tree climbers.

In primitive and remote areas, assume that bears are present; in more developed sites, ask the park staff about the current bear situation. Most encounters are food related, as bears have an exceptional sense of smell and will eat anything. A clean site combined with care and caution will keep these foragers away from your campsite. Store all food, cooking equipment, and garbage in tightly sealed containers and place well away from your tent. In remote areas or those with recent bear activity, store all items in storage lockers or bear canisters, or suspend them in a sack 12 feet above the ground, 6 feet below branches, and 12 feet from neighboring trees. Make sure that your site is clean and never leave food unattended. Clean utensils and cooking equipment at least 100 feet from your site, and never dump uneaten food on the ground. Do not bring food into your tent, and do not sleep in clothes worn while preparing food. Never leave scented products of any kind—food, beverages, or personal-care products such as lotion or sunscreen—in your vehicle unattended in the park area. Generally, proper food preparation and garbage disposal will help maintain a pristine wilderness, the safety of bears and other wildlife, and an enjoyable camping experience for everyone.

RATTLESNAKES

New York has a variety of snakes—including garter, milk, and water snakes—most of which are benign. Timber rattlesnakes, northern copperheads, and eastern massasauga rattlesnakes are the exceptions, though they primarily dwell in very isolated areas. According to the DEC, the massasauga is found in two isolated marshy areas: one near Syracuse and the other near Rochester. The copperhead is found mostly along the Hudson Valley but is mostly absent from the Catskills. Timber rattlesnakes are the most widely dispersed of the three and are found in rugged deciduous forests along the southern edge of the state and up into the eastern Adirondacks. Encounters with any of these species are very rare.

When hiking, stick to well-used trails and wear over-the-ankle boots and loose-fitting long pants. Rattlesnakes like to bask in the sun and won't bite unless threatened. Do not step or put your hands where you cannot see, and avoid wandering around in the dark. Step on logs and rocks, never over them, and be especially careful when climbing rocks or gathering firewood. Always avoid walking through dense brush or willow thickets. Keep in mind that rattlers want to avoid confrontation and generally will alert you if you wander too close for their comfort. Hibernation season is October through April.

The only known treatment for a snakebite is intravenous antivenom, only available at a hospital. If you are hiking alone and get bitten, calmly walk to where you can get help. If someone in your group has been bitten, send another person to get help quickly while the victim rests.

MOSQUITOES

You will encounter mosquitoes on most of the hikes described in this book. Insect repellent and/or repellent-impregnated clothing are the only simple methods to ward off these pests. Mosquitoes in New York are known to carry the West Nile virus, so all due caution should be taken to avoid mosquito bites.

Black Flies

Though certainly a pest and maddening annoyance, the worst a black fly will cause is an itchy welt. They are most active from mid-May through June, during the day, and especially before thunderstorms, as well as during the morning and evening hours. Insect repellent has some effect, though the only way to keep them from swarming is to keep moving.

Ticks

Ticks are often found on brush and tall grass, waiting to hitch a ride on a warm-blooded passerby. Adult ticks are most active in New York between April and May and again between October and November. Among the local varieties of ticks, the black-legged tick, commonly called the deer tick, is the primary carrier of Lyme disease. Several strategies reduce the chances of ticks getting under your skin. Some people choose to wear light-colored clothing, so ticks can be spotted before they make it to the skin. Most important, be sure to visually check your hair, back of neck, armpits, and socks at the end of the hike. During your post-hike shower, take a moment to do a more complete body check. For ticks that are already embedded, grasp the tick as close to the skin's surface as possible with tweezers, and pull upward with steady, even pressure. Do not puncture a tick, as this might release harmful bacteria. Use disinfectant solution on the wound.

Poison Ivy, Oak, and Sumac

Recognizing and avoiding poison ivy, oak, and sumac are the most effective ways to prevent the painful, itchy rashes associated with these plants. Poison ivy occurs as a vine or ground cover, 3 leaflets to a leaf; poison oak occurs as either a vine or shrub, also with 3 leaflets;

COMMON POISONOUS PLANTS

POISON SUMAC

POISON OAK

POISON IVY

and poison sumac flourishes in swampland, each leaf having 7 to 13 leaflets. Urushiol, the oil in the sap of these plants, is responsible for the rash. Within 14 hours of exposure, raised lines and/or blisters will appear on the affected area, accompanied by a terrible itch. Refrain from scratching because bacteria under your fingernails can cause an infection. Wash and dry the rash thoroughly, applying a calamine lotion to help dry out the rash. If itching or blistering is severe, seek medical attention. If you do come into contact with one of these plants, remember that oil-contaminated clothes, pets, or gear can easily cause an irritating rash on you or someone else, so wash not only any exposed parts of your body but also clothes, gear, and pets, if applicable.

Hunting

UNLIKE MANY NATIONAL AND STATE PARKS, HUNTING IS ALLOWED in Adirondack Park. Separate rules, regulations, and licenses govern the various hunting types and related seasons. Though there are generally no problems, hikers may wish to forgo their trips during the big-game seasons, when the woods suddenly seem filled with orange and camouflage. The following is a list of big-game seasons.

- **EARLY BEAR SEASON**: The first Saturday after the second Monday in September; lasts four weeks

- **ARCHERY SEASON** (deer and bear): September 27 to opening of regular season

- **MUZZLE LOADING SEASON**: Seven days prior to regular season

- **REGULAR SEASON**: Next-to-last Saturday in October through the first Sunday in December

Tips on Enjoying Adirondack Park

ONE OF THE BEST FEATURES OF ADIRONDACK PARK IS its democratic nature. It is meant for the public to enjoy its wild character and is open to all. There are few if any fees, permits, or licenses required for this enjoyment—and none for those who simply wish to hike the trails. Simply drive to your trailhead, get out of your car, and hit the trail. It is a luxury and a responsibility. Without park staff cleaning, maintaining, and policing the way they typically do in other parks, the burden for cleanliness, maintenance, and your own safety lies on your own shoulders. Practicing the ethos of carry-in and carry-out will ensure that other hikers enjoy the wilderness as much as, and in the same way, you have. By maintaining campsites, lean-tos, and fire rings, you will ensure others get to enjoy them and find them useful too. Avoiding destructive behavior, such as chopping down trees for firewood or causing unnecessary erosion by taking shortcuts, means the forever-wild character of the Adirondacks will remain.

Backcountry Advice and DEC Regulations

THE ENTIRE PARK LIES UNDER THE JURISDICTION OF THE DEC, and its rules and regulations regarding hiking and backcountry camping apply for all state lands within the park. Camping is permitted within the forest preserve without a permit as long as you follow the regulations below. The DEC's rules and regulations are essentially the same sound, safe, and practical advice I would offer, so I recap them below.

- CAMPING IS PROHIBITED WITHIN 150 FEET OF ANY ROAD, trail, spring, stream, pond, or other body of water, except at areas designated by a CAMP HERE disk.

- GROUPS OF 10 OR MORE PERSONS OR stays of more than three days in one place require a permit from the New York State Forest Ranger responsible for the area.

- LEAN-TOS ARE AVAILABLE IN MANY AREAS ON A FIRST-COME, first-serve basis. Lean-tos cannot be used exclusively and must be shared with other campers.

- USE PIT PRIVIES PROVIDED NEAR POPULAR CAMPING AREAS and trailheads. If none are available, dispose of human waste by digging a hole 6 to 8 inches deep at least 150 feet from water or campsites. Cover with leaves and soil.

- DO NOT USE SOAP TO WASH YOURSELF, clothing, or dishes within 150 feet of water.

- DRINKING AND COOKING WATER SHOULD BE BOILED for five minutes, treated with purifying tablets, or filtered through a filtration device to prevent instances of giardia infection.

- FIRES SHOULD BE BUILT IN EXISTING FIRE PITS OR FIRE-PLACES if provided. Use only dead and down wood for fires. Cutting standing trees is prohibited. Extinguish all fires with water, and stir ashes until they are cold to the touch. Do not build fires in areas marked by a NO FIRES disk. Camp stoves are safer, more efficient, and cleaner.

- CARRY OUT WHAT YOU CARRY IN. Practice "leave no trace" camping and hiking.

- KEEP YOUR PET UNDER CONTROL. Restrain it on a leash when others approach. Collect and bury droppings away from water, trails, and campsites. Keep your pet away from drinking-water sources.

- OBSERVE AND ENJOY WILDLIFE AND PLANTS, but leave them undisturbed.

- REMOVING PLANTS, ROCKS, FOSSILS, OR ARTIFACTS from state land without a permit is illegal.

- EXCEPT IN AN EMERGENCY, or between December 15 and April 30, camping is prohibited above an elevation of 4,000 feet in the Adirondacks.

- AT ALL TIMES, ONLY EMERGENCY FIRES ARE PERMITTED above 4,000 feet in the Adirondacks.

Trail Etiquette

WHETHER YOU'RE ON A CITY, COUNTY, STATE, OR NATIONAL PARK TRAIL, always remember that great care and resources (from nature as well as from your tax dollars) have gone into creating these trails. Treat the trail, wildlife, and fellow hikers with respect.

- HIKE ON OPEN TRAILS ONLY. Respect trail and road closures (ask if not sure), avoid possible trespassing on private land, and obtain all permits and authorization as required. Also, leave gates as you found them or as marked.

- LEAVE ONLY FOOTPRINTS. Be sensitive to the ground beneath you. Stay on existing trails rather than blazing new ones. Pack out what you pack in. No one likes to see the trash someone else has left behind.

- NEVER SPOOK ANIMALS. An unannounced approach, a sudden movement, or a loud noise startles most animals. Surprised animals can be dangerous to you, to others, and to themselves. Give them extra room and time to adjust to your presence.

- OBSERVE THE YIELD SIGNS that are displayed around the region's trailheads and backcountry. They advise that hikers yield to horses, and bikers yield to both horses and hikers. A common courtesy on hills is that hikers and bikers yield to any uphill traffic.

- WHEN ENCOUNTERING MOUNTED RIDERS OR HORSE PACKERS, hikers can courteously step off the trail, on the downhill side, if possible. Speak to the riders before they reach you and do not hide behind trees. You are less spooky if the horse can see and hear you. Resist the urge to pet or touch the horses unless you are invited to do so.

- **PLAN AHEAD.** Know your equipment, your ability, and the area in which you are hiking—and prepare accordingly. Be self-sufficient at all times; carry necessary supplies for changes in weather or other conditions. A well-executed trip is satisfying.

- **BE COURTEOUS TO OTHER HIKERS, BIKERS, EQUESTRIANS,** and others you encounter on the trails.

West–Central Hikes (1-7)

N

0   5   10
miles

Dun Brook Mountain

Sabael

Indian Lake

Snowy Mountain

Speculator

Hamilton Mountain

W. Branch Sacandaga River

30

Blue Mountain Lake

30

30

Wakely Mountain

Pillsbury Mountain

8

Piseco

Piseco Lake

7

Raquette Lake

Raquette Lake

S. Branch Moose River

6

Grass Mountain

Hoffmeister

Hamilton County
Herkimer County

2

4

3

Fourth Lake

ADIRONDACK STATE PARK

28

Old Forge

8

Stillwater Reservoir

Stillwater Mountain

Independence River

Stone Dam Mountain

1

Oneida County

Herkimer County
Lewis County

Woodgate

28

Otter Creek

Moose River

12

5

12

Black River

Booneville

1

PART ONE
West-Central Hikes

1 Bear and Woodhull Lakes

SCENERY: ✿ ✿ ✿
TRAIL CONDITION: ✿ ✿ ✿
CHILDREN: ✿ ✿
DIFFICULTY: ✿ ✿ ✿
SOLITUDE: ✿ ✿ ✿ ✿

DISTANCE: *10.2 miles; 1.2-mile side trip*
HIKING TIME: *5–7 hours*
OUTSTANDING FEATURES: *Lakeside hiking, side trip to broad waterfall*

More than half of the loop to Bear and Woodhull lakes includes gravel and dirt access roads, but these roads are closed to traffic or are lightly traveled. The trail portions are truly excellent and include two lakes, a pond, and seasonal streams to hike beside. A side trip to Remsen Falls is easily accessible along the loop as well. The Remsen Falls side trip is wheelchair accessible, with a special parking area located closer to the falls.

🚶🚶 The trail network in the Woodhull Lake area is bisected by a gravel road that provides access to several designated roadside campsites as well as the wheelchair-accessible Remsen Falls picnic and camping area. If camping is part of your agenda, you may want to consider the roadside sites or backpack to the lean-to and designated sites by Woodhull Lake. Camping in other areas is permitted as long as you follow the basic backcountry camping guidelines laid out by the DEC. The best parking is available in the McKeever parking area at the end of McKeever Spur Road. I found that hiking counterclockwise around the loop brings you into the wilderness soonest and leaves the easier roadside hiking for the return trip.

From the parking area, head southeast along the gravel road past the barrier gate. The road climbs gently but is free of obstruction, so you quickly cover the first 0.7 miles and reach the first designated campsite. You pass a second campsite within a couple hundred feet, a bridge at 0.8 miles, and yet another campsite at 1.1 miles. You reach the beginning of the foot trail on your right at 1.3 miles. The foot trail has a sign indicating that to your right are Bear Lake, 1.7 miles,

1 Bear and Woodhull Lakes

N

0   0.5   1
mile

Woodhull Lake

Big Woodhull-Sand Lake Falls Trail

lean-to

Bloodsucker Pond

Moose River

Remsen Falls

fire pit

Remsen Falls Trail

McKeever-Bear Lake-Woodhull Trail

Nicks Lake Trail

S. Branch Administrative Rd.

Wolf Lake Landing Rd.

saddle

waterfall

Bear Lake

Bear Lake Trail

Moose River

ADIRONDACK STATE PARK

BLACK RIVER WILD FOREST

Brewer Lake

P

McKeever Rd.

28

Moose River Rd.

28

and Bear Creek parking area, 8.8 miles. Continuing straight, you reach Remsen Falls in 2.4 miles, Woodhull Mountain in 6.9 miles, and Woodhull lean-to in 4.6 miles. This intersection is immediately before another bridge.

Head south, to your right, on the blue-marked trail toward Bear Lake. The trail immediately traverses a flat, wet section that could easily swallow a boot or two. The trail climbs more than 300 feet over the next 0.5 miles through the familiar birch, beech, and maple forest of the western Adirondacks. You reach the crest of your climb at 1.9 miles in a saddle between two hills, where you begin to catch glimpses of Bear Lake in front of you. The view is heavily obscured by the forest canopy but promises a picturesque destination. As you weave your way down the next 0.5 miles to the lake, steep ledges become exposed on your left. More than 40 feet high in sections, the ledges reinforce the rugged wilderness feel that hikers so frequently seek along the myriad trails of the Adirondacks. Depending on the season and water level, you might be privy to a tiny waterfall cascading along these ledges around 2.3 miles. Certainly not a frothing cascade, the rivulet breaks through a cleft in the ledge and is

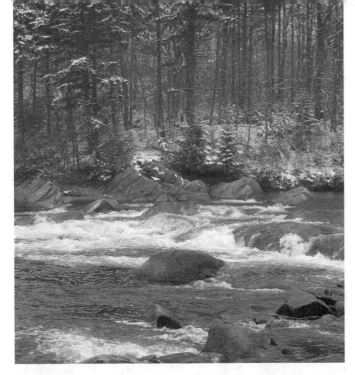

Remsen Falls

undoubtedly seasonal in nature. The trail's descent ends abruptly on the shores of Bear Lake, which is admirably framed before you by a large black cherry tree. A little farther along the trail is an abandoned fire ring, where more exceptional views of the lake await you.

The trail winds its way along the northern and then eastern shore of Bear Lake for the next 0.3 miles, where you encounter a feeder stream. After rock-hopping across the stream, you will find a trail intersection on the opposing shore. Continuing straight along a blue-marked trail would bring you to Nejeer Hill Trail at 1.9 miles and the Bear Creek parking area at 6.9 miles. To your left and marked in yellow are the Woodhull lean-to, 2.4 miles, and Remsen

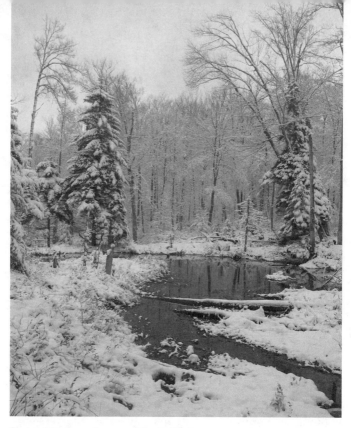

Seasonal stream on the way to Woodhull Lake

Falls, 5.2 miles. Continue to your left eastward along the yellow-marked trail.

The trail parallels the stream for the next 0.3 miles, providing a pleasant waterscape as you begin to climb away from Bear Lake. While traversing this section of the trail, I encountered several different colors of flagging tape riddled with notes. Because it was hunting season, I first suspected that it was the work of hunters trying to retrace their steps. After a while, the magnitude of the flagging and the consistent spacing showed that it was instead the work of rescue crews trying to find a lost hunter. Every year, hunters and some hikers get lost in the woods, and many are not found. Upon returning to civilization, I learned that this case had a happy ending, as the hunter was found miles away after spending two cold November nights alone in the woods. Not all are as fortunate, and it is a stark reminder that communicating your plans and having regular check-ins are essential.

As you near the crest of your climb, 4.3 miles, the trail swings southward. This southern jog of 0.4 miles brings you close to shores of Bloodsucker Pond, a small pond fed by a stream from Woodhull Lake. When you reach the pond and stream, 4.7 miles, the trail swings east again, and the stream accompanies you as you head east another 0.1 mile to a major trail intersection. To your right is a series of trails that takes you deeper into the Black River Wild Forest as well as to our major destination, the Woodhull lean-to, at 0.3 miles. To your left are the return leg of the loop with Remsen Falls, 2.5 miles away, and the McKeever parking area, 5.4 miles away. To reach the lean-to, turn right and head over the bridge into the giant mire, where the trail to the lean-to, marked in red, diverges to your left from the other trails that delve into the Black River Wild Forest. The trail down to the lean-to is basically a long mire, so expect to be nimble and inevitably end up with muddy boots anyway. As you near the lean-to, you first notice a pit toilet and, if you're anything like me, can't help but wonder if future routes might avoid long mires that end at toilets. Regardless of your musings on trail routing, you reach the large lean-to on Woodhull Lake shortly after, 5 miles. The lean-to has obviously been worked on recently and is the equivalent of two lean-tos. Situated within 10 feet of the shore, it has excellent views and is a great stopping point. But be forewarned, it is a popular destination and, due to its proximity to the road, likely occupied. Return through the mire to the intersection encountered before the bridge to continue along the loop, 5.2 miles from the start.

Heading north from the intersection, you will follow red snow-mobile markers and quickly reach a vehicle barrier gate. The road you intersect continues to the right down to Wolf Lake Landing, but you will be heading north, to your left, toward Remsen Falls. You pass several campsites as you head north 1.1 miles along the road to the next major intersection. This intersection is just past two closely spaced campsites and is marked by a trail sign. The designated parking area for the wheelchair-access road to Remsen Falls is also located at this intersection. To the right is Remsen Falls, 0.6 miles, while continuing along the main access road to your left takes you back to the McKeever parking area in 3 miles. Even if you don't plan to take the side trip to Remsen Falls, a more pleasant return leg is along the red-marked trail.

Continue to your right along the wheelchair-access road, marked in red, another 0.1 mile, where you reach another intersection. To your right is Woodhull Mountain, 4.5 miles; straight ahead is Remsen Falls, 0.5 miles; and to your left is the return trip to the McKeever parking area, 3.1 miles.

SIDE TRIP TO REMSEN FALLS
(mileage along loop does not include this 1.2-mile trip)

The side trip to Remsen Falls adds 1.2 miles to your total trip, but because it follows wheelchair-accessible paths, this diversion takes little time and effort. Heading almost due north along the wide, flat, and sandy access path, you quickly reach Moose River just above the falls. You can see a lean-to on the opposing shore, and you find a fire pit, picnic table, and designated camping area at the end of the trail. Continue along well-worn paths past the picnic table to get farther downriver to view the falls. When you reach a second picnic table, the falls are clearly visible. Less of a falls and more of a broad rapid, the tumble of water drowns out most surrounding sounds. Another fire pit is located farther downstream if you desire more privacy. Return the way you came to complete the loop.

Back on the main trail, head west along the dirt access road, marked in red. This access road is closed to vehicles, though you might see mountain bikers, as this is a popular biking area. The return trip is mostly level and easygoing and passes without incident. You pass a large culvert at 8 miles, Bear Lake Trail on your left at 8.9 miles, a second culvert at 9.1 miles, and a trail register at 9.8 miles. This second register seems to be used primarily by people visiting the falls or heading straight to the mountain. Head past the barrier gate where there is a large turnaround, and continue west to the McKeever parking area for a total trip length of 10.2 miles, 11.4 including the side trip.

DIRECTIONS: From NY 28, turn east onto McKeever Road, 16.2 miles northeast of the intersection of NY 12 and NY 28 in Alder Creek or 10.4 miles southwest of Old Forge. Continue to your right onto McKeever Spur Road at 0.3 miles, past an old railroad station. Continue another 0.4 miles. The parking area is on your right and marked with DEC signs.

GPS Trailhead Coordinates	1 Bear and Woodhull Lakes
UTM Zone (WGS 84):	18T
Easting:	0492667.9
Northing:	4828613.8
Latitude:	N 43° 36' 44.92"
Longitude:	W 75° 05' 25.72"

2 Black Bear Mountain

SCENERY: ✿ ✿ ✿ ✿	DISTANCE: *4.9 miles*
TRAIL CONDITION: ✿ ✿	HIKING TIME: *3 hours*
CHILDREN: ✿ ✿ ✿ ✿	OUTSTANDING FEATURES: *Bald mountain,*
DIFFICULTY: ✿ ✿	*scenic views*
SOLITUDE: ✿ ✿ ✿	

A popular destination in summer and fall, this tiny peak provides excellent views of the Fulton Chain of Lakes. It is a great choice for children and beginner hikers, but if you wish for solitude, then plan to go during the off-season, especially winter.

From the southeast corner of the parking area, head south, paralleling the road. After passing a deteriorating concrete bridge on your left, you will quickly reach a sign indicating the trailhead to your left. The trail register is just inside the tree line. The trail—marked in yellow hiking, ski, and biking disks—heads northeast through mixed hardwoods. Approximately 0.3 miles in, a stream becomes visible on your left. At 0.7 miles, you reach the intersection with the return leg of the trip on your right. This trail, also marked in yellow, is a more direct and steeper ascent to the peak, but returning along this trail provides some great views along the descent.

To make the longer and more scenic loop, continue northeast along the left fork through some muddy sections. At approximately 1 mile, you reach a clearing encircled by small firs with rock cairns marking the path. Shortly after, you cross a couple of streams over log-and-plank bridges and will soon see the mountain looming off to your right. The grade along the north side of the mountain is relatively flat, and you soon reach another trail intersection, which is a little less than the halfway point, 2.3 miles. To your left are Uncas Trail, 0.6 miles, and Uncas Road parking area, 1.5 miles. To your right are the summit, 0.5 miles, and the return to NY 28, 2.6 miles.

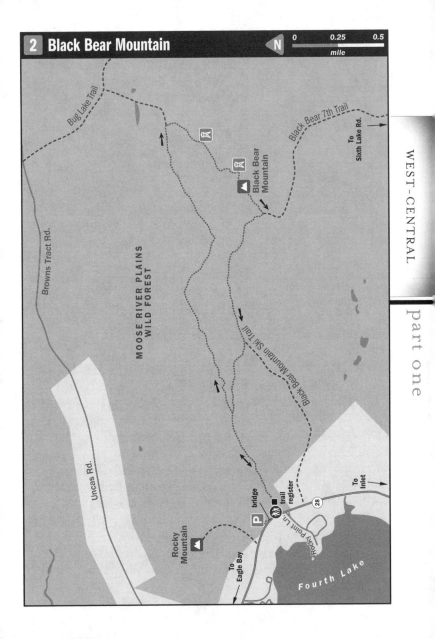

Bug Lake Trail

Black Bear 7th Trail

To
Sixth Lake Rd.

Black Bear Mountain

Browns Tract Rd.

MOOSE RIVER PLAINS
WILD FOREST

Black Bear Mountain Ski Trail

Uncas Rd.

Rocky
Mountain

bridge

trail
register

P

28

To
Inlet

To
Eagle Bay

Rocky Point Ln.

Fourth Lake

The trail begins to climb immediately, and the forest transitions from maple and beech to evergreens fairly quickly. A quarter mile from the intersection, 2.5 miles from the start, you reach an opening in the evergreens and a lookout on your left. From here you have an excellent view of Seventh Lake, part of the Fulton Chain of Lakes.

The Fulton Chain is a series of connected lakes that begins at Old Forge Pond and ends with Eighth Lake. It is a popular destination for a wide variety of boaters and is the beginning of the North Forest Canoe Trail. In fact, First through Fifth lakes comprise an unbroken length of 14 miles. A series of channels separates Old Forge Pond and Sixth through Eighth lakes from this main expanse. The connection of these lakes was part of steamboat inventor Robert Fulton's vision of an Adirondack Canal. Although the canal was never built, the chain still bears Fulton's name.

Returning to the trail, the path winds in and out of stands of evergreens and over large spans of open ledge. At 2.8 miles, the trail runs into a four-foot ledge that you navigate to reveal another opening in the canopy and yet another lookout on your left. Head

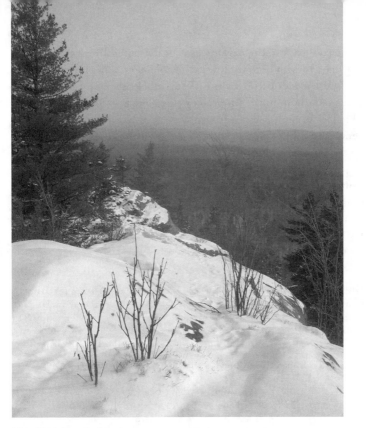

Near Black Bear Peak

northeast into the dense evergreens to find the yellow-marked trail that quickly leads you to the actual summit about 0.1 mile ahead. The actual summit is hard to distinguish along the mostly flat, bald peak, but a series of small ledges to the left of the trail makes an excellent spot to dangle your feet and enjoy the view. To the south, you can see portions of the town of Inlet as well as Sixth and Seventh lakes. To the west, you can make out portions of Fourth Lake.

The trail back to the parking area heads generally west but is now mostly marked with blue trail disks. The descent is steeper than the ascent but provides better views of Fourth Lake than any of the lookouts or even the summit. After you weave your way down the many small ledges some 0.4 miles from the peak, the trail levels off, and you encounter a few more wet areas. At 3.7 miles, the blue markers begin to thin, and yellow markers become more prevalent. After a short jog where the trail swings northward, the return trail parallels the inbound trail awhile and, after descending along a broad road, you reach the first intersection at 4.2 miles. Hike the remaining 0.7 miles back to NY 28 and the parking area for a total trip length of 4.9 miles.

DIRECTIONS: Coming from the west, head east 1.2 miles from the junction of Big Moose Road and NY 28 in Eagle Bay. The spacious parking lot is on your left. From the east, head north 0.9 miles from Inlet, along NY 28, and look for the parking area on your right. There are two entrances, so if you miss the first in either direction, simply enter the second.

GPS Trailhead Coordinates	2 Black Bear Mountain
UTM Zone (WGS 84):	18T
Easting:	0516511.0
Northing:	4845503.7
Latitude:	N 43° 45' 51.86"
Longitude:	W 74° 47' 40.15"

3 Bubb, Sis, and Moss Lakes

SCENERY: ✿ ✿ ✿	SOLITUDE: ✿ ✿
TRAIL CONDITION: ✿ ✿ ✿ ✿ ✿	DISTANCE: *7 miles*
CHILDREN: ✿ ✿ ✿ ✿ ✿	HIKING TIME: *3–4 hours*
DIFFICULTY: ✿	OUTSTANDING FEATURES: *Lakeside hiking*

These three pristine lakes offer a variety of activities and feature trails with varied levels of accessibility, making this an ideal trip for the entire family. The Moss Lake circuit, with its broad, flat trails and wheelchair-accessible sections, provides an excellent opportunity for the very young—or those no longer interested in hiking rugged trails—to enjoy the beauty of the Adirondacks. On the other hand, the Bubb and Sis lakes section features rugged trails and remote lakes that are easily combined with the circuit for extended and more invigorating trips.

🚶🚶 There are a variety of ways to explore these pristine lakes. The Moss Lake circuit has long sections that are wheelchair accessible, and the majority of the trail is flat, broad, and easy to navigate. Two larger parking areas are also available near Moss Lake along Big Moose Road (also known as County Road 1). These parking areas should be used for extended stays, end-to-end hikes, and day use in the Moss Lake area because the Bubb and Sis parking area can realistically accommodate only five to six vehicles, two of which are handicapped spaces. You can make it an end-to-end hike if you start at the Bubb and Sis trailhead along NY 28 and get picked up or meet at one of the Moss Lake parking areas along Big Moose Road. The trip described here includes taking a straight route past Bubb and Sis lakes, then following the circuit around Moss Lake, and finally returning along the straight route between Bubb and Sis lakes.

The trail, marked with yellow disks, begins in the northwest corner of the small parking area along NY 28. The trail climbs immediately, and after a few dozen yards, you reach the trail register. The

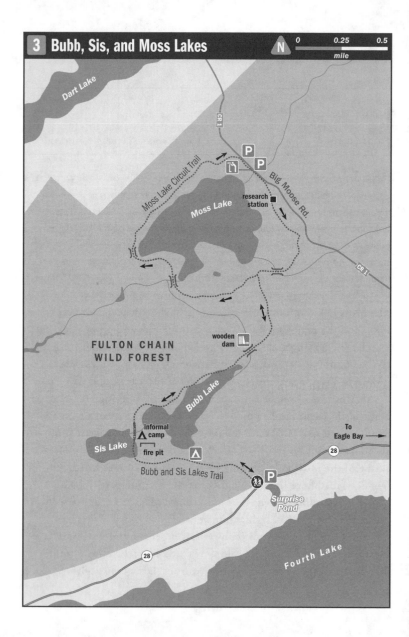

N

0   0.25   0.5
mile

Dart Lake

CR 1

P P

Moss Lake Circuit Trail

Moss Lake

Big Moose Rd

research station

CR 1

FULTON CHAIN WILD FOREST

wooden dam

Bubb Lake

Sis Lake

informal camp

fire pit

Bubb and Sis Lakes Trail

To Eagle Bay

28

Surprise Pond

28

Fourth Lake

trail then swings northward with a steep incline, and you quickly reach the intersection with the Vista Trail, marked in blue, on your left. Continue straight ahead and the trail soon levels off. The trail is mostly level from this point on, and within 0.5 miles of the start, Bubb Lake comes into view. You encounter a minor fork in the trail just before the lakeshore. To the left is the main trail, while straight ahead are an excellent point from which to view the lake and a designated campsite nestled off to the right of the short path that leads to the lake.

Continuing to the left along the main trail, you'll cross a small stream as you skirt the southern edge of Bubb Lake. Within minutes, you'll reach a stand of hemlocks along the edge of Sis Lake. In the height of summer, this is a very tranquil area, and the calls of loons can be heard throughout. From this grove of hemlocks, the trail swings northward and passes an informal campsite on your left. This site has benches, a fire pit, and an informal path that follows the western edge of Bubb Lake. Just past this site is a boardwalk, 0.8 miles, which crosses the small wetland between the two lakes.

Once on the opposite shore, the trail swings eastward and follows the northern shore of Bubb Lake. After 0.8 miles, you reach the

Moss Lake

northeastern tip of the lake and encounter yet another heavily used area to the right of the trail. There are several fishing regulation signs, and a bit farther east off the trail is a fire pit. The main trail veers to the left of this heavily used area, and at 1.6 miles, you cross a small stream over a log-and-plank bridge and notice a wooden dam on the left. The trail becomes broader after this crossing and soon swings northward as it heads to the Moss Lake circuit, which you reach at 2.3 miles. To the right is the most direct route to the parking areas along Big Moose Road and the day-use areas around the lake. Turn left and head clock-wise around the circuit.

The trail around Moss Lake is broad and sandy and easily accom-modates two or more abreast. It is a popular circuit for groups of walkers, so don't expect much solitude. The lake is hidden from view until you reach a bridge that crosses a stream and wetland that sprawls out to the west. Climb a short hill, and wind your way northward along the western edge of the lake. At mile 3.1, you'll cross another log-and-plank bridge; shortly after, the trail swings northeast. As you near the eastern edge of the lake, you pass a road that intersects the trail on the left, 3.7 miles, and head into the day-use area of the lake. Dotting the eastern shore are myriad paths, picnic areas, and designated campsites, as well as an observation deck, that are more easily explored than described. The circuit path bypasses most of these areas and soon reaches the first of two parking areas. At the second parking area is a trail register, campsite register, historical information placard, and a map of the circuit and campsites.

Continuing along the main circuit, you'll pass side trails leading to a couple of campsites on your right and then enter an open field with a research station with tall fences off to left. At 4.3 miles, you pass a side trail to the left that leads to Big Moose Road and shortly after, another bridge that crosses Moss Lake's main inlet stream. You soon reach the intersection with the Bubb and Sis lakes trail, 4.7 miles. Return the way you came for a total trip of 7 miles.

DIRECTIONS: *Sis and Bubb lakes parking area*   From the hardware store in Old Forge, head east 7.9 miles along NY 28; the parking area is on the left. From the intersection of CR 1/Big Moose Road and NY 28 in Eagle Bay, head east 1.4 miles along NY 28; the parking area is on your right.

Moss Lake parking area   From the intersection of CR 1/Big Moose Road and NY 28 in Eagle Bay, head north 2.2 miles on CR 1/Big Moose Road; the large parking area is on your left.

GPS Trailhead Coordinates	3 Bubb, Sis, and Moss Lakes
UTM Zone (WGS 84):	18T
Easting:	0512523.2
Northing:	4845719.6
Latitude:	N 43° 45' 58.91"
Longitude:	W 74° 50' 39.89"

4 Cascade Lake

SCENERY: ☆ ☆ ☆ ☆	DISTANCE: *5.9 miles*
TRAIL CONDITION: ☆ ☆ ☆ ☆	HIKING TIME: *3–4 hours*
CHILDREN: ☆ ☆ ☆ ☆	OUTSTANDING FEATURES: *Lakeside hiking,*
DIFFICULTY: ☆	*tall waterfall, historic site*
SOLITUDE: ☆ ☆ ☆ ☆	

Not to be confused with Cascade Lake in the High Peaks region, this scenic loop in the town of Inlet offers an excellent trip around the lake and includes a 43-foot waterfall. The roughly 6-mile circuit follows old access roads that are wide enough for two to walk side by side nearly the entire way. Excellent camping spots are found along the north shore.

The trailhead is located in the southeast corner of the spacious parking area along Big Moose Road. A painted map of the Pigeon Lake Wilderness trail system is also located next to the trail register. The trail briefly parallels the road in a southeasterly direction before swinging east under the canopy of pole-size hardwoods. Trail markers switch between yellow cross-country skiing and red foot-trail disks. Because most of the trail is along old access roads, it would be hard to lose your way. The roads once led to Camp Cascade, originally a summer camp for Charles E. Snyder that easily could have been considered one of the "Great Camps." It was later sold at a fraction of the asking price to Dr. George Longstaff. Longstaff, already an owner of a sailing camp on nearby Moss Lake, transformed the property to an all-boys equestrian camp. When the camp began to falter during World War II, it became coed. The state acquired the property in 1962 and had plans to build a campground, but shortly afterward removed the buildings in accordance with the Forever Wild initiative.

About 0.3 miles in, you intersect this old road and begin to head northeast. As it was in the past, the broad road is clearly used

4 **Cascade Lake**

N

| 0 | 0.25 | 0.5 |

mile

Cascade Falls

Uncas Rd.

Cascade Mountain

road begins

fireplace

clearing

overgrown asphalt

Sucker Brook

Cascade Lake

stone retaining wall

South Shore Trail

Eagle Creek

Cascade Lake Link Trail

steel bridge

ADIRONDACK STATE PARK

PIGEON LAKE WILDERNESS

Chain Ponds Trail

Cascade Lake Trail

To Eagle Bay

Big Moose Rd.

by horses in the summer (watch your step) and would make an excellent skiing trail in the winter. Numerous wet spots dot the road but are easily bypassed along the shoulders. At 1 mile, the road intersects the south-shore trail on your right. Though the south-shore trail parallels the lake's southern shore, you will not be able to see the lake until you reach the eastern tip near the waterfall. However, the circuit seems to make the most sense hiked in a counterclockwise direction, so mileage and directions are given accordingly.

The forest matures as you head farther along the trail, and two can walk easily abreast for almost the entire circuit. A few mucky areas sprawl across the trail during the next couple of miles, but overall it is a very pleasant woodland walk. At 2.5 miles, you catch your first glimpse of the lake as the forest becomes thicker with evergreens. Roughly 3 miles from the parking area, you come across an open meadow with a stream cutting its way westward to Cascade Lake. Head a brief distance east into the surrounding forest, along any of the numerous footpaths, to find the namesake waterfall. The narrow cascade falls 43 feet onto the rocks below before trickling out into the meadow. To the right of the falls is a path that climbs through

Cascade Falls in the height of the summer

a narrow passage to the top. The plateau of bedrock at the top is an excellent spot to sit and enjoy the falls.

Continuing along the loop, the trail quickly reaches a long wet and muddy section. Stay on the path and pick your footing carefully, as the broad marshland will quickly suck the ill-placed foot knee-deep into the muck. As I can attest, you will likely have to wait until you reach the lakeshore, almost 0.5 miles ahead, before you can wash off the black muck. Upon reentering the woods, the trail weaves uphill briefly before joining the north-shore road at 3.3 miles. The north-shore road drops down to the lake at 3.5 miles and skirts it fairly closely for the next mile with excellent views of the water as well as a few remnants of the abandoned girls camp. The first relic is an old stone fireplace and foundation approximately 0.1 mile after reaching the lake. Small hardwood saplings are starting to reclaim this clearing and many of the other sites farther along. The camp stopped operating in the 1950s and was acquired by the state in 1962, so the regenerative growth is an excellent example of how quickly nature reasserts itself. The next clearing has a thick carpet of ferns with dense eastern white pine regeneration that will quickly close in the open space. The most striking reestablishment is at 3.8 miles, where an old tennis court is being broken up and covered by a carpet of grass to the left of the trail. Saplings form a thicket around this formerly impervious surface, and you can tell that it won't be long before roots begin to assist the grasses in breaking up the surface.

Many of these clearings would make excellent campsites, but the more popular ones, found farther along, have better views of the lake. None of the sites are designated (they're often referred to as informal sites), so DEC regulations dictate that you must be 150 feet from both the lake and the trail. One such grassy location is found near the lakeshore a little past the tennis court. Probably the most desirable and likely occupied lakeside campsite is found at 4 miles. An old stone retaining wall holds back the forest on your right, while a heavily shaded lawn sprawls out on your left. The parklike setting is an obvious destination, and its proximity to the road means that weekend campers likely pack in far more than the backcountry camper could. Shortly after, you leave the shores of the lake and come to a fork in the trail. A trail to the right, 4.5 miles from the start, heads to Chain Ponds, Queer Lake, Chub Pond, and the rest of the Pigeon Lake Wilderness. Continue straight ahead 0.1 mile to a short steel bridge that crosses the outlet of Cascade Lake. A broad,

Old stone fireplace along the north shore trail

picturesque wetland sprawls out on your right, and you notice substantial beaver activity in the vicinity. Immediately after, you will pass through another clearing to the left of the trail and quickly reach the intersection with the south-shore trail. From here, it is another mile back to the parking area.

DIRECTIONS: From NY 28 in Eagle Bay, head north on CR 1/Big Moose Road. The spacious parking lot is 1.3 miles on the right.

GPS Trailhead Coordinates	4 Cascade Lake
UTM Zone (WGS 84):	18T
Easting:	0513533.2
Northing:	4847612.6
Latitude:	N 43° 46' 53.20"
Longitude:	W 74° 49' 54.54"

5 Gleasmans Falls

SCENERY: 🐾 🐾 🐾	DISTANCE: *5.8 miles*
TRAIL CONDITION: 🐾 🐾 🐾 🐾	HIKING TIME: *2–3 hours*
CHILDREN: 🐾 🐾 🐾 🐾	OUTSTANDING FEATURES: *Beaver dam,*
DIFFICULTY: 🐾 🐾	*series of small waterfalls cascading in a narrow gorge*
SOLITUDE: 🐾 🐾 🐾 🐾	

This relatively level out–and–back hike is a great trip for hikers who like to arrive at a beautiful destination. The falls roar through a narrow gorge, and you can view this torrent from high atop the gorge's sheer walls. Another unique feature is a close–up view of an old beaver dam along the trail. Situated on the western fringe of the park boundary, it is less frequented and offers a good chance for solitude.

🚶🚶 After driving up the long, bumpy road, you will already feel removed from the rest of the world. Indeed, finding the parking area among the unnamed roads will likely be the hardest aspect of this clearly defined trail. You will be following the Beach Mill Pond Trail, which provides access to a more extensive trail system in the Independence River Wild Forest. From the parking area, you walk down a gravelly path to an open and grassy area with a winding tannin-laden creek. Burnt Creek is the outflow of the previously dammed Beach Mill Pond, where a sawmill once produced lumber. You will have to negotiate a few small muddy spots on the way to a recently constructed wooden footbridge. On the other side of the bridge, you will enter the forest again, where tall pines and hemlocks shade the trail thoroughly. The trail, emblazoned with yellow DEC trail markers, is wide and clearly visible among the leaf and needle litter. With few obstructions and roots, typical of most Adirondack trails, the trail is very easygoing. At 0.2 miles, you will pass the trail register, and the forest transitions from mostly conifers to mixed hardwoods. Interspersed with the dominant beech and maple trees

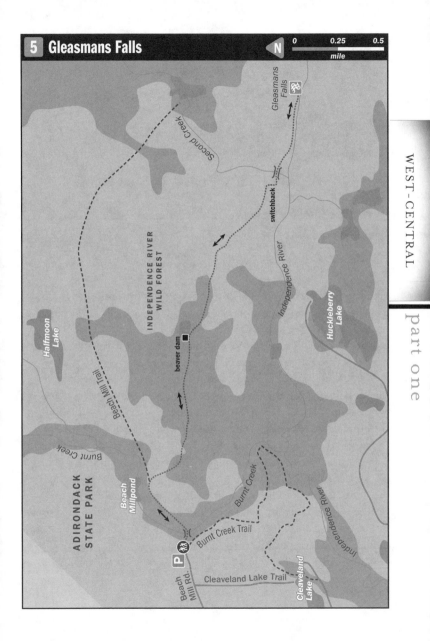

N

0   0.25   0.5

mile

ADIRONDACK
STATE PARK

INDEPENDENCE RIVER
WILD FOREST

Halfmoon
Lake

Second Creek

Gleasmans Falls

switchback

Independence River

Huckleberry
Lake

Beach Mill Trail

Burnt Creek

beaver dam

Beach
Millpond

Burnt Creek Trail

Burnt Creek

Cleaveland Lake Trail

Cleaveland
Lake

Independence River

Beach Mill Rd.

P

are large cherry trees, all of which provide a dense and high canopy. The ground cover is mostly trout lily, and the lack of saplings or brush provides deep views into the surrounding forest. The trail meanders north briefly, and you glimpse Beach Mill Pond off to your left through a dense stand of hemlocks.

At 1.6 miles, you come to the outflow of an old beaver dam. Planks laid lengthwise help you traverse a few muddy spots and are followed by a log-and-plank bridge. After crossing the bridge, the trail immediately turns east to skirt the edge of the beaver pond. A section of the dam has been breached, so the water is not as high as it might have been. The skeletons of pine trees left standing in what is now less a pond and more a marshland provide a stark contrast to the dense forest that sits atop a slight ridge to your right. You will find some good birding and aquatic wildlife viewing in this area, but I doubt that you will linger long, as mosquitoes and black flies relish in ambushing curious hikers here. The muddiest area of the trail is along this edge, and because the slight ridge restricts the trail, your options for avoiding the muck are limited.

After leaving the beaver dam area, the trail passes through a small meadow and then rises to a more scrubby area, where the canopy is significantly more open and lower. This brief foray into an open hilltop setting adds a nice variety to the trail's ecological niches. After hopping over a few narrow seasonal creeks, the trail transitions back to a dense forest where pines are the dominant species. At 2.3 miles, the trail has a small switchback that descends to the confluence of Second Creek and the boulder-strewn Independence River. Another recently constructed log-and-plank bridge crosses Second Creek, after which the trail climbs slightly over a small hillock dotted with large moss-covered boulders and then descends to Independence River.

The first of the series of falls is visible here, and a slight scramble to the river's rocky banks will give some glimpses of the falls upriver. You begin to view the roaring falls from atop the narrow gorge after passing a fire pit and informal campsite. These dramatic views of the rushing waters are the true reward for the hiker and are especially powerful during the spring melts. None of the falls is very tall, but the channeling of the river through this narrow gorge, combined with huge boulders, creates a beautiful scene of cascading and foaming waters. As the trail continues to climb the cliffs along the side of the river, the views become more panoramic, with several spectacular views straight down the sheer gorge walls onto the falls. Indeed, the views get successively better along the trail, so do not stop until the trail turns north back into the forest around 3 miles. The trail eventually winds back to the river, but the falls will be behind you at this point, and only a scramble back along the rocky wash above the falls will provide any views.

DIRECTIONS: From NY 12/NY 26/South State Street in Lowville, take County Road 22/River Road until it turns into CR 26/Number Four Road. Turn right onto Loson Road, and then take a quick right onto McPhilmy Road at 0.4 miles. After crossing Erie Canal Road at 2.5 miles, continue on McPhilmy 0.3 miles, and then take a left onto the unmarked Beach Mill Road. Continue on the rough and bumpy Beach Mill Road, bearing left at the fork, until the road ends, 3 miles.

GPS Trailhead Coordinates	5 Gleasmans Falls
UTM Zone (WGS 84):	18T
Easting:	0477784.1
Northing:	4850588.5
Latitude:	N 43° 48' 28.13"
Longitude:	W 75° 16' 28.20"

6 Mitchell Ponds

SCENERY: ✿ ✿ ✿	SOLITUDE: ✿ ✿ ✿ ✿
TRAIL CONDITION: ✿ ✿ ✿ ✿	DISTANCE: *5.6 miles*
CHILDREN: ✿ ✿ ✿ ✿ ✿	HIKING TIME: *2–3 hours*
DIFFICULTY: ✿ ✿	OUTSTANDING FEATURES: *Lakeside hiking*

Nestled in the middle of the Moose River Plains Wild Forest, the trail to Mitchell Ponds is an easy stroll along an old logging road, followed by a quick jaunt along the lake. The trail follows mostly level ground and is easy to follow, so expect to make good time. Trail conditions also make it an excellent introduction to hiking.

🚶🚶 To reach Mitchell Ponds, you have to enter the Moose River Plains Wild Forest. Purchased in 1963 from the Gould Paper Company, the 50,000-acre block is bisected by a network of rough roads and myriad roadside campsites, more than 170 mostly primitive sites. The roads are gravelly and filled with potholes and other hazards characteristic of lightly maintained backwoods roads, so a four-wheel-drive, high-clearance vehicle is recommended. Registration booths are at the entrances to the area, and the whole road system is open to vehicles from Memorial Day to the end of hunting season. It is a very popular destination during hunting season, and you might think that more vehicles are in the recreation area than on the main roads.

The parking area is essentially an access road, but room for a handful of vehicles is on either side of the road. The trail, marked with yellow disks, is a continuation of this access road and heads nearly due west. After a few hundred feet, you pass a barrier gate. The trail is mostly level, and because it is an old access road, you can easily walk two abreast. The trail is free from obstructions, so you can easily observe the surrounding landscape as you make good time along the road. At 1.4 miles, you will see a small stream and wetland on the left, though most of the trip is through dense woods.

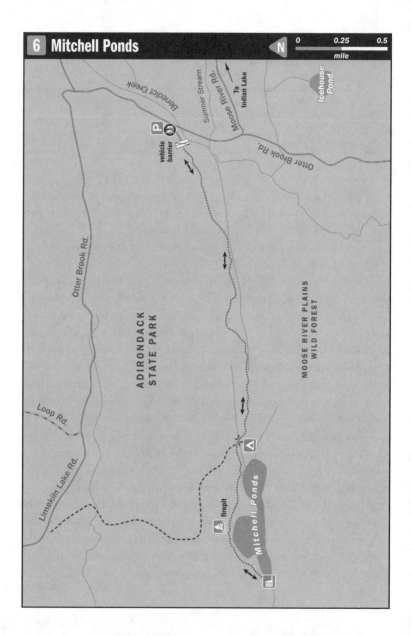

N

| 0 | 0.25 | 0.5 |
mile

Icehouse Pond

Benedict Creek

Sumner Stream

Moose River Rd.

To Indian Lake

Otter Brook Rd.

P

vehicle barrier

Otter Brook Rd.

Loop Rd.

Limekiln Lake Rd.

ADIRONDACK STATE PARK

MOOSE RIVER PLAINS WILD FOREST

firepit

Mitchell Ponds

At 1.8 miles, you reach a clearing and a fork in the trail. Straight ahead is a designated campsite on the eastern tip of Mitchell Ponds. It has a picnic table and excellent views of the water, making it an ideal stopping point even if you don't plan to camp.

Back at the intersection, the trail continues to your right through a very wet section and over a deteriorating bridge. Just on the other side of the bridge is a second intersection on your left. Straight ahead is the trail that leads to the north access point on Moose River Road, while the trail along the shores of Mitchell Ponds is on your left. From this point on, the path is no longer a wide forest road but a typical Adirondack foot trail. The trail weaves along Mitchell Ponds's northern shore, providing excellent views and a tranquil setting. At 2.2 miles, you reach an old fire pit in the midst of the trail and an old sign reminding you of the carry-in, carry-out policy that is in place for the entire Adirondack Park. Past the fire pit, the trail becomes more rugged, narrower, and a little harder to make out but nothing that exceeds the skills of even novice hikers.

Shortly after the fire pit, the trail swings southwest as it weaves its way to the western tip of the ponds. A jumble of boulders fills the

Beaver dam on west end of Mitchell Ponds

steep hillside to your right, forming many small caves and crevices. At 2.8 miles, you reach this tip and the end of the trail, where a beaver dam blocks the outflow of the pond. You can get a few views back on the ponds from the large rocks, but crossing the outlet would probably be wet and difficult. Return the way you came for a round-trip of 5.6 miles.

DIRECTIONS: *From the west vehicle entrance near Limekiln Lake* From the registration booth, follow Moose River Road east and south 7.9 miles. The parking area is on your right.

From the east vehicle entrance near Wakely Dam on Cedar River Road From the registration booth, follow Moose River Road west 10.3 miles, 0.3 miles past the Otter Brook Road junction. The parking area is on your left.

GPS Trailhead Coordinates	6 Mitchell Ponds
UTM Zone (WGS 84):	18T
Easting:	0523493.8
Northing:	4835759.1
Latitude:	N 43° 40' 35.33"
Longitude:	W 74° 42' 29.37"

WEST-CENTRAL

part one

7 Panther Mountain and Echo Cliffs

SCENERY: ✿ ✿ ✿ ✿ ✿
TRAIL CONDITION: ✿ ✿ ✿ ✿
CHILDREN: ✿ ✿ ✿ ✿ ✿
DIFFICULTY: ✿ ✿

SOLITUDE: ✿ ✿
DISTANCE: *1.4 miles*
HIKING TIME: *1.5 hours*
OUTSTANDING FEATURES: *Panoramic views*

Definitely the shortest trail described in this book, Panther Mountain and Echo Cliffs are not short on scenery. With less than a mile to the scenic lookout, hikers are quickly rewarded with panoramic views of Piseco Lake. The scenic vista, combined with some stunning cliffs beside the trail, makes it an excellent excursion in one short package. Its popularity in the summer attests to its beauty, so plan on going in the off-season or early morning hours to avoid the crowds.

🚶 Parking for the Panther Mountain and Echo Cliffs trail is on the eastern side of County Road 24, just south of the entrance to Little Sand Point Campground. Piseco Lake actually has three campgrounds along its shores; I recommend *The Best in Tent Camping: New York State* for further descriptions of the campgrounds. Located on the boundary between the West-Central and Southern regions and fairly close to the Central Region, Piseco Lake makes a great base camp to explore the Adirondack foothills.

Though the trail is often described as Panther Mountain, your actual destination is the ledge along Echo Cliffs. The ledge is 2,420 feet in elevation, 300 feet less than the Panther Mountain summit. The mountain apparently got its name from the abundance of mountain lions, or panthers, in the area in the early 1800s. The town board of Arietta consequently offered a bounty of $20 to purge the area of panthers in 1837. Also known as cougars, the large predators have been absent from New York and the Adirondacks since the 1800s. Rumors abound regarding recent sightings throughout the Adirondacks, and the rumor mill has gone so far as to claim that the DEC is releasing cougars

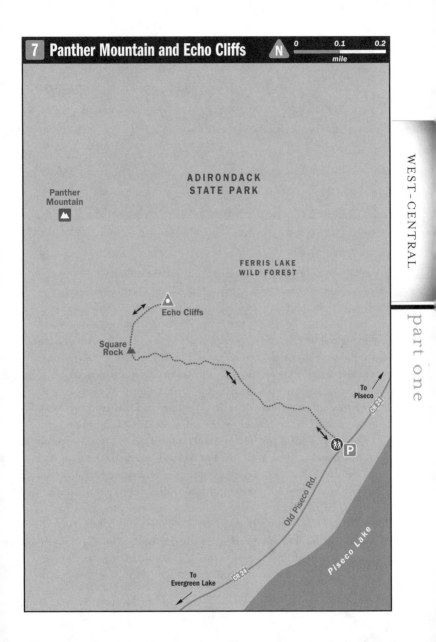

ADIRONDACK
STATE PARK

Panther
Mountain

FERRIS LAKE
WILD FOREST

Echo Cliffs

Square
Rock

To
Piseco

CR 24

Old Piseco Rd.

CR 23

Piseco Lake

To
Evergreen Lake

WEST-CENTRAL

part one

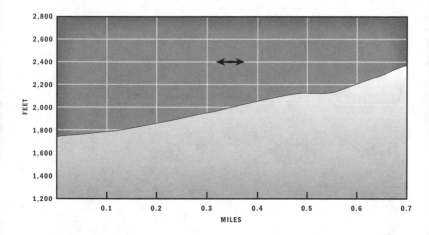

to curtail the deer population. The rumors have spread wildly through online chat rooms and even sprouted YouTube videos suggesting a conspiracy. The DEC has refuted the claims numerous times and even created a Web page to clarify the issue. The official stance is that a self-sustaining population of cougars does not exist in New York, that sightings are almost always cases of mistaken identity, and that the extremely rare actual cougars are escapees or releases from private owners.

The parking area is a long pulloff that is about 50 yards long and could easily accommodate dozens of vehicles. A DEC trail sign with a blue disk marks the trailhead on the opposite side of the road.

This trail is ideal for novice hikers, children, or simply a quick climb for a scenic view. Well worn and clearly marked, the path is easy to follow. Its short, steep section is a simple reminder of the rewards hiking offers. The trail, marked with blue disks, is obviously popular; heavy use has turned the path into a wide swath along the forest floor. Under the dense canopy of birch, maple, and beech trees, the trail is mostly level as you head generally northwest, but it gradually becomes steeper after you pass through a jumble of angular boulders and begin to head west. Approximately 0.6 miles in, you pass a large

View of Piseco Lake from Echo Cliffs

square boulder on your left. After the square boulder, the trail turns northward, and you soon pass under sheer rock walls to your left. The trail is much steeper along this section, but the climb is brief, and after you pick your way up the roots of a hemlock tree that grows on the right side of the trail, you are rewarded with views of Piseco Lake. The lookout is the top of Echo Cliffs, and while the summit of Panther Mountain is behind you to the northwest, no clear path leads to it. The long, exposed outcrop provides a panoramic view of most of Piseco Lake, including Higgins Bay and Spy Lake to the east and directly across the lake, as well as portions of Irondequoit Bay, Big Bay, and the Piseco outlet to the south.

DIRECTIONS: *From the east* From NY 8, turn left onto CR 24/West Shore Road, 19.4 miles east of the intersection of NY 8 and NY 365 in Cold Brook. Continue 2.6 miles, and look for the pulloff on your right. If you reach Little Sand Point Campground, you are 0.5 miles too far north.

From the west From NY 8, turn right onto CR 24/West Shore Road, 8.8 miles east of the intersection of NY 8 and NY 30 in Speculator. Follow West Shore Road around the northern tip of Piseco Lake, and look for the parking area on your left, 0.5 miles south of Little Sand Point Campground, 5.4 miles along CR 24/West Shore Road.

GPS Trailhead Coordinates	7 Panther Mountain and Echo Cliffs
UTM Zone (WGS 84):	18T
Easting:	0535811.4
Northing:	4806595.5
Latitude:	N 43° 24' 41.00"
Longitude:	W 74° 33' 27.65"

Square boulder along path

Central Hikes (8-15)

0   5   10
miles

Saratoga County

Essex County
Warren County

Lake George

Schroon Lake

87

9   Hoffman Mountain

Schroon Lake

87   Schroon River

9

Schroon
Lake

12

Pottersville   9

The Glen   28

Hudson River

8

Minerva

28N   North Creek   Baldhead Mountain

Boreas River

Hudson River   Bakers Mills

9   13   ADIRONDACK STATE PARK   15

28   14

8

Warren County
Hamilton County   8

11

Dun Brook Mountain   Indian Lake   30   Wells   30

Sabael   Indian Lake

Snowy Mountain   Speculator

30   Lake Pleasant

Blue Mountain Lake   Sacandaga Lake   Hamilton Mountain

30   Pillsbury Mountain

28   Wakely Mountain   8

Piseco   Piseco Lake

Raquette Lake   Grass Mountain

Raquette Lake   Hoffmeister

2

PART TWO
Central Hikes

8 Auger Falls

SCENERY: ✿ ✿ ✿ ✿	DISTANCE: *1.1 miles*
TRAIL CONDITION: ✿ ✿ ✿ ✿	HIKING TIME: *1 hour*
CHILDREN: ✿ ✿ ✿ ✿ ✿	OUTSTANDING FEATURES: *Spectacular*
DIFFICULTY: ✿	*waterfall, riverside stroll*
SOLITUDE: ✿ ✿ ✿	

The powerful falls on the West Branch of the Sacandaga River are truly a sight to see. Channeled into a narrow flume, the river plunges 40 feet in a torrent of foamy waters. As a short-distance loop, this is an excellent introductory hike for children, but take caution near the falls because the cliffs are steep and potentially slippery.

🚶🚶 It is easier on your car, as well as logistically, to park in the large lot that is straight ahead after turning off NY 30. Consequently, directions and mileage are from this point rather than the parking area down the bumpy access road, which is closer to the foot trail's start. From the main parking area, head back toward NY 30, and turn left down the access road. Continue down the bumpy and rutted dirt road until you see the DEC trail sign on your left at 0.3 miles. The trail register is a short distance down the foot trail.

Some people may scoff at the need to sign in for such a short trail, but I encourage hikers to sign in on this and every hike. The DEC and the state base many of their trail-maintenance and funding decisions on trail registers. If you want to see your favorite trails maintained or want more like them, then let the registers act as your democratic voice in the wilderness.

On the trail, walk along the rolling terrain a little more than 0.3 miles through mixed hardwoods. Ahead, you will begin to hear the roar of the falls, and it is likely that you will abandon the trail to explore the numerous paths that diverge from the main trail to find the best vantage point. Many of the paths that offer excellent

CENTRAL

part two

Sacandaga River

Macomber Creek

P

30
8

To
Lake
Pleasant

**ADIRONDACK
STATE PARK**

**SIAMESE PONDS
WILDERNESS**

Sacandaga River

P

trail
register

stone
fireplace

Auger
Falls

30
8

To
Wells

views and photos of the torrential falls are worn and crumbling, so watch your step. The most dramatic part of the waterfall occurs where the river is channeled into a cataract and then plunges down into the gorge formed by the sheer walls of the river. The cliffs on the opposite shore are spectacular, and the dwarfed trees clinging to its ledges only add to the sense of wildness. Photo-worthy views of the opposing sheer cliff and waterfall are found below the falls. Indeed, you can easily reach the middle of the river by hopping along the large boulders that are strewn about at the outwash of the falls. Huge trees lie tangled among the boulders, and it is not hard to picture the powerful flow of water hurling boulders and trees about. To relocate the trail, head back toward the top of the falls, and you will eventually see the yellow disks that mark the trail. It will take you to a beautiful exposed portion of ledge that sits atop the cataract, where an old fireplace has been partially demolished. This spot marks the halfway point and makes an excellent place to stop, with the falls thundering below.

To complete the loop, head upstream along the worn but unmarked path. Dense conifers crowd the trail in many locations, and

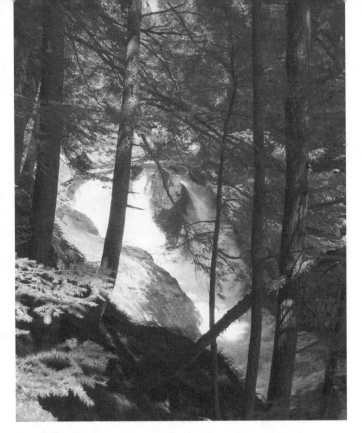

Auger Falls

you often have to skirt or climb over fallen trees. The calm waters of the river above the falls are a striking contrast to the turbulent waters below. Keep an eye out for a wooden footbridge on the opposite shore, as this indicates that you are nearing the point to turn back toward the parking area. When you reach a sandy beach near a broad, flat calm in the river, climb over the hillock to your left and you will come out on the northern end of the parking area.

DIRECTIONS: From the intersection of County Road 17 and NY 30 in Wells, head north on NY 30/NY 8. At 3.3 miles, bear left to stay on NY 30. At 1.8 miles, turn right onto the gravel drive that leads to the parking area. The drive is unmarked and comes up on you quickly, with few places to turn around if you miss it, so slow down on NY 30. Parking is available straight ahead in a large gravel lot or at the trailhead immediately to your right down a bumpy dirt road. The road is part of the loop, and the end of the trail is the parking lot, so there is no mileage difference where you park.

GPS Trailhead Coordinates	8 Auger Falls
UTM Zone (WGS 84):	18T
Easting:	0560580.9
Northing:	4813025.2
Latitude:	N 43° 28' 4.00"
Longitude:	W 74° 14' 59.08"

9 Blue Ledges

SCENERY: ✿ ✿ ✿ ✿	DISTANCE: *5 miles*
TRAIL CONDITION: ✿ ✿ ✿ ✿	HIKING TIME: *2–3 hours*
CHILDREN: ✿ ✿ ✿ ✿	OUTSTANDING FEATURES: *Vertical cliffs in*
DIFFICULTY: ✿ ✿ ✿	*the Hudson River Gorge*
SOLITUDE: ✿ ✿ ✿ ✿	

The beautiful stroll through a deep forest would be excuse enough to go on this hike, but the spectacular cliffs and sandy beaches in the Hudson River Gorge elevate it to a don't-miss list. In the height of summer, it makes an excellent picnic or swimming destination with the option for excellent riverside camping. On dam-release days, especially during spring and fall, you will likely see rafters and kayakers navigating the turbulent rapids that flow at the base of these gigantic cliffs.

🖈 The trail, marked with blue disks, begins across the road from the parking area on the left. You will immediately cross a stream over a log-and-plank bridge. Shortly after, you come to a very mucky area with the trail register in the middle of the mire. The trail heads westward to the shore of Huntley Pond, where you have to pick your way through mud and tangles of roots. The walk along the shoreline requires a good deal of rock- and root-hopping to stay out of the muck, but this is very brief and followed by a slight climb into the hardwood forest.

At 0.5 miles, you pass between two large moss-covered boulders and then descend 0.3 miles down to a stream. After crossing the stream, the trail levels off, and you hike mostly on flat terrain. This level portion of the trail continues approximately 0.8 miles and is very easygoing. The high canopy allows deep views into the forest on your left, while broad openings along the meandering stream to your right provide a stark contrast. You will likely notice some very large eastern white pines interspersed with birch and maple trees. At 1.5 miles, you

begin a 0.5-mile climb up the hill, whose contour you have been following since the stream crossing. As you climb southward, larger pine
trees loom along the trail, and you will hear the Hudson's rushing
waters to your right. Despite how close the thundering rapids seem just
beyond the tree line, you will not be able to see the river until you reach
the trail's end. At 2 miles, you cross a large exposed portion of ledge,
which marks the beginning of the descent to the river. This lookout
reveals nothing through the thick foliage of summer, but when the
leaves fall, it promises excellent views. The last half mile of the trail is
the steepest section but is easily managed on both the descent and the
return climb. The eastern white pines sporadically encountered along
the trail earlier now dominate the forest as you reach the riverbank.

You see glimpses of the ledges through the evergreen canopy, but
the scale of the cliffs is not apparent until you reach the end of the
trail. As you emerge directly on the riverbank, the Blue Ledges loom
300 feet on the opposite shore.

The vertical wall of rock draped by pines and cedars, seen across
the broad river, makes a dramatic and peaceful setting. Paths leading both up- and downriver explore the riverbank and take you to

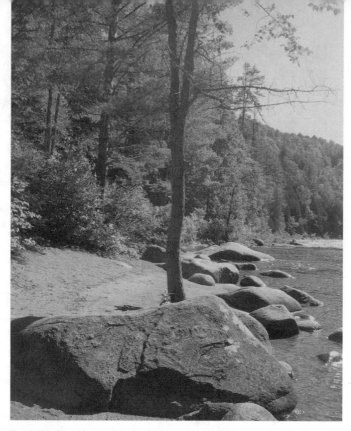

Sandy beach at the end of the trail

several sandy beaches. High water during spring and fall makes for whirlpools and rapids that are best observed or rafted with commercial outfitters. During periods of lower water in the summer, sheltered areas provide a good opportunity for swimming. If you choose to swim, be mindful that the river still has a powerful current and that dam releases from Lake Abanakee on Tuesdays,

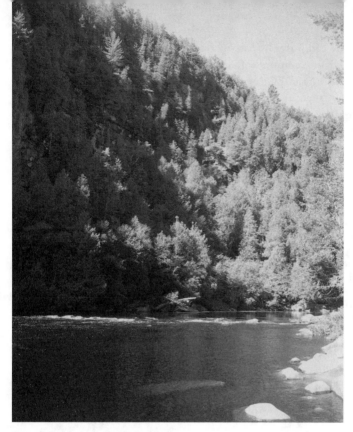

Steep cliffs seen across the Hudson River

Thursdays, Saturdays, and Sundays raise the river by two feet. Upstream and around the bend is one major rapid, while downstream are some major Class IV and V rapids. These rapids are visible from the trail's end and provide a popular amusement shortly after midday on dam-release days. Designated riverside camping areas are also downstream near these treacherous rapids. You can reach the campsites by passing through a thicket of brush near the river's edge. Camping is limited to these areas, and they seem to fill up. Otherwise, DEC regulations require backpackers to set up camp at least 150 feet from any body of water. The Hudson River Gorge is an exceptionally beautiful destination in the Adirondacks, and unless you are willing to raft down the river, this trail is virtually the only way to see its beauty.

DIRECTIONS: Heading north along NY 28 N from Minerva, turn left onto North Woods Club Road. The turn is more like bearing left, but it is located along a curve and hill, so you will likely miss it heading south along NY 28 N. The dirt road is smooth and accessible for most vehicles. At 3.7 miles, you cross the Boreas River and see designated roadside camping on both sides of the road. The road climbs steeply afterward. As it descends, the trail sign is visible on the left at 6.7 miles. The parking area along North Woods Club Road could accommodate close to a dozen vehicles if parked close together and perpendicular to the road.

GPS Trailhead Coordinates	9 Blue Ledges
UTM Zone (WGS 84):	18T
Easting:	0571676
Northing:	4853679
Latitude:	N 43° 49' 57.79"
Longitude:	W 74° 06' 30.58"

10 Castle Rock

SCENERY: ⛺ ⛺ ⛺ ⛺	DISTANCE: *3.7 miles*
TRAIL CONDITION: ⛺ ⛺ ⛺	HIKING TIME: *2 hours*
CHILDREN: ⛺ ⛺ ⛺ ⛺	OUTSTANDING FEATURES: *Interesting rock*
DIFFICULTY: ⛺ ⛺	*formations, lookout on lake*
SOLITUDE: ⛺ ⛺ ⛺ ⛺	

From a glance at a map, this trail looks deceptively uninteresting, but it has a lot to keep your interest. The analogy to a castle is well founded, and those with active imaginations will find themselves naming gates, turrets, and other structures while exploring the area. As a short loop, it provides a refreshing change from the innumerable out-and-backs typical of summits and other trails in the park.

👣 The parking area is a small pulloff near the Minnowbrook Conference Center. The trail register is just up the road within sight of the sandy parking area. However, the trail does not begin until a little more than 0.3 miles down the road. Mileage given here is from the trail register. Follow the private gravel road, and bear right where the conference center driveway rejoins the road. Red trail markers on the right tell you to bear right at the next fork in the road.

At 0.3 miles, you will finally reach the trail on your right. On your left is a stream, which is the outlet of Chub Pond, as it flows to Blue Mountain Lake. Shortly after the trail portion starts, you come to a log bridge crossing this stream and a fork in the trail. To your left is the south route to Castle Rock, while to your right is Upper Sargent Pond and the north route. Cross the bridge to follow the south route, a rolling trail through mixed hardwoods. Yellow disks emblazon the trail, and at 0.6 miles, you can see Chub Pond and a broad wetland to your right. The view is limited, but better views of the pond are available on the return trip along the northern route. When I hiked the trail, rain had been falling sporadically for days, so the trail was very wet; in fact it was basically a stream in some sections

(particularly on the northern route). But judging by the number of mucky spots, it is safe to say that this trail is typically wet.

The trail is a deep-woods walk among tall hemlock, birch, maple, and spruce trees. The landscape is dotted with large, mossy boulders that hint at the large rock faces to come. At 0.8 miles, you will find a small dip, as well as a fork, in the trail; 0.3 miles to your left is Blue Mountain Lake, while Castle Rock is 0.7 miles to your right. After crossing a small brook, the trail begins to climb steadily. Openings in the forest canopy indicate that the lake sprawls off to your left, but you cannot see it until you reach the summit.

At 1.2 miles, you come to what I imagine to be the castle's gates. The base of the large granite outcrop towers above you on your right, with a narrow passage between it and some of the boulders that lie among the cliff's talus. Running water babbles underneath the sheer castle wall, sparking images of activities on the other side. Paths that eventually lead back to the main trail weave through the maze of boulders, providing excellent opportunities for exploration.

Back along the trail, a brief climb brings you to the intersection of the northern route, on your left. The climb to Castle Rock's final

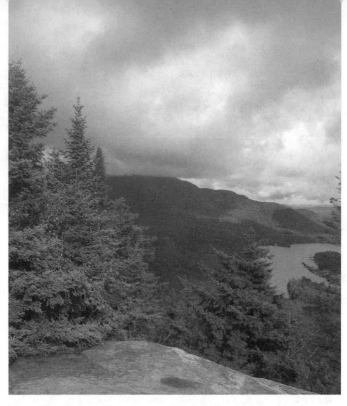

View of Blue Mountain Lake from atop Castle Rock

lookout is on your right, through spruces and paper birches. You reach the summit as you squeeze through another narrow passage. Climbing atop the rock ledge on your left reveals excellent views of the tree-covered mountains to the north. While this view is beautiful and panoramic, the real gem is the view from atop the ledge, or rather the southern turret, on your right. Sitting 700 feet above Blue Mountain Lake, this sheer cliff provides excellent panoramas of the wooded islands that dot the lake. The cliff's sheer walls and the way it

Bridge that connects the southern and northern routes

juts out above the tree line invoke the feeling of being atop a lookout tower and, in combination with the "gate" at the base, gives rise to the impression of a castle. Take caution around the cliff edge during wet or icy conditions.

Returning along the northern route, the trail is less steep and descends gradually with numerous stream crossings. This portion is marked with red DEC disks and is easy to follow. At 1.9 miles, you cross a stream and come to a fork in the trail; the Upper Sargent

Pond Trail heads off to your left, while to the right is the return to the trailhead and parking area. While the southern route definitely has some wet areas, the northern route has notably more and longer mucky spots. The forest matures as you descend, and you rock-hop across multiple streams that flow to your right. At 2.3 miles, you come to a meadow, where the sound of water rushing to your right is much more distinct. The trail flattens out a bit more, and the mucky areas become more frequent. You encounter Chub Pond again at 2.8 miles, with views of Castle Rock through the hemlocks that surround the wetland. Multiple vantage points of the pond are available along the trail, and shortly you come back to the juncture where the log bridge crosses the outlet of Chub Pond. The stroll back to the parking area passes quickly along the flat roads.

DIRECTIONS: From the intersection of NY 28/30/28 N in Blue Mountain Lake village, head north on NY 30/28 N. Turn left onto Maple Lodge Road at 0.6 miles. Continue on Maple Lodge Road 1.7 miles until you see the trail register, and park at the pulloff on the left side of the road before the Minnowbrook Conference Center.

GPS Parking Area Coordinates	10 Castle Rock
UTM Zone (WGS 84):	18T
Easting:	0544142.5
Northing:	4857899.8
Latitude:	N 43° 52' 21.62"
Longitude:	W 74° 27' 4.95"

SCENERY: ✿ ✿ ✿ ✿	DISTANCE: *2.2 miles*
TRAIL CONDITION: ✿ ✿ ✿ ✿	HIKING TIME: *1 hour*
CHILDREN: ✿ ✿ ✿ ✿	OUTSTANDING FEATURES: *Interesting*
DIFFICULTY: ✿ ✿	*geological formations*
SOLITUDE: ✿ ✿ ✿	

In a region noted for beautiful lakes and panoramic mountains, this geological oddity adds a spectacular variation. Formed over millennia, Chimney Mountain provides a great opportunity to view the geological forces that shaped the Adirondacks. Exploring the numerous formations will occupy most for hours, but for the spelunker and ama-teur geologist, a day trip probably will not suffice.

🕱 The parking area for Chimney Mountain, as well as Puffer Pond and Kings Flow East trails, is on private land with a day-use fee of $2 per car. Many of the Adirondack Park's best hikes and features are available through cooperation between private landholders and the DEC. To ensure this cooperation and to encourage future col-laborations, please respect private property and pay the day-use fee.

To reach the trailhead and register, walk up the gravel drive past several cabins, approximately 0.2 miles from the parking area. The register is located beneath the shade of the encompassing forest. The Puffer Pond and Kings Flow East trailheads are to your right, while the Chimney Mountain Trail is to your left. Trail maps often show the two sharing a section of the trail, but the portion shared is actu-ally the access road before the trail register. Mileage given is from the actual trailhead and not from the parking area or trail register.

Passing through a thick band of saplings along the forest's edge, you will quickly notice that the trail is wide, well worn, and easy to fol-low. Blue DEC disks mark the trail but are hardly necessary except near the top, where numerous paths lead to caves and other geological points

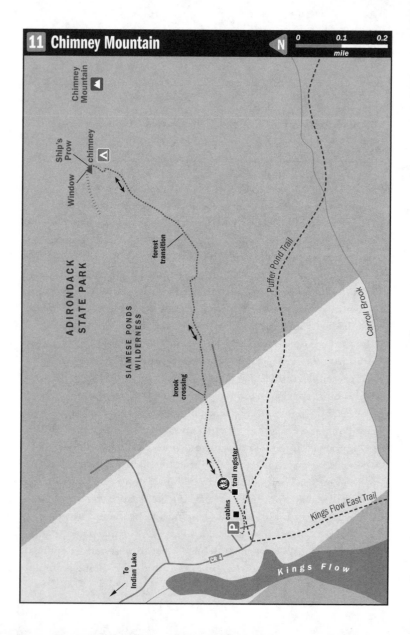

11 Chimney Mountain

N

| 0 | 0.1 | 0.2 |

mile

Chimney Mountain

Ship's Prow

Window

chimney

ADIRONDACK STATE PARK

SIAMESE PONDS WILDERNESS

forest transition

brook crossing

trail register

P cabins

Puffer Pond Trail

Carroll Brook

Kings Flow East Trail

To Indian Lake

CR 4

Kings Flow

of interest. Shrouded in tall hardwoods, most notably birches and maples, the trail is fairly level until 0.2 miles, where you cross a brook and the climbing begins. The grade is moderate at first but steadily increases toward the peak. The forest eventually transitions from the deep woodlands to a more open and parklike setting approximately 0.7 miles along. On steeper sections of the trail, take a look back and you will see Round Lake, which seems to hover at the bases of Crotched Pond Mountain and Kunjamuk Mountain.

Closer to the summit, you will begin encountering informal paths that wind off to your left. This maze of paths leads to some lesser rock formations, to numerous crevices and caves, and to another elevated ridge from which you can look back at the chimney. The caves have precipitous drops, so be cautious when off the main trail, especially with curious and bold children. Exploring the caves should be left to people who are properly experienced and equipped. Do not attempt these activities if you are a novice. However, there are plenty of wonders and much to explore along the main trail, so don't feel like you are missing out if you do not explore off the trail.

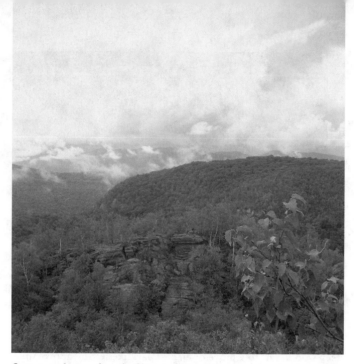
Opposing ridge seen from the Chimney

The spire, an amalgamation of metamorphosed rocks, will begin to tower ahead and draw you through ledges that flank the trail. The marked trail ends here, but do not let that stop you from scrambling among the rocks. Just be cautious near the northern edge, as the drop-off is precipitous. The convoluted layers of different materials will likely raise an eyebrow as you puzzle over how such rocks come into being. See page 1 for an elementary description. The story of these epoch transformations is revealed in the exposed portions of Chimney Mountain.

A description of all the interesting formations and ways to find and explore them all is beyond the scope of this book and, frankly, this author. However, I will name a couple that you can easily and

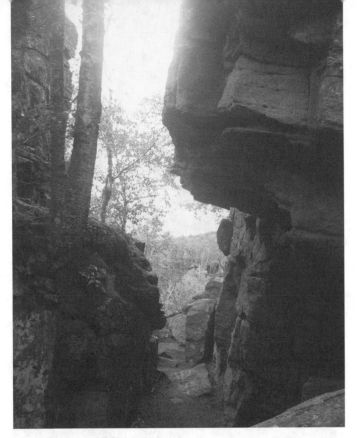

Passage between rock formations

safely access from the main trail. The main passage you encounter has the jumble of rocks that make up the Chimney to your left and a narrow ledge called the Ship's Prow. The prow is easily walkable, but it narrows and the fall is more precipitous as you go—know your limits before attempting to walk to its end. Turning left at the trail's end, you walk under a striking overhang and come out with the Chimney looming to your right. Climbing along its base to the opposite side

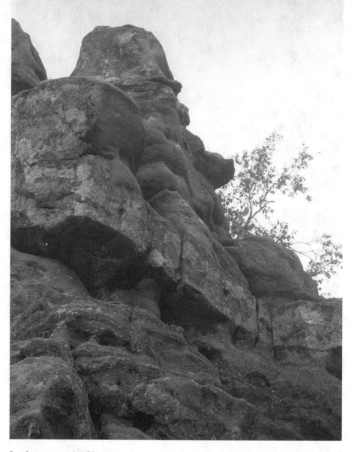

Looking up at the Chimney

will reveal the Window; it frames the western ledge and is easy to crawl into. In addition to the formations, various points offer panoramic views of the ridge to the west, as well as seemingly endless peaks in every direction.

Chances are that as you looked up onto the spire when you climbed, you missed a path to the right, which leads to an informal campsite. As you leave the Chimney, this path is more obvious off to your left. Just past the campsite, the path leads not only to the actual summit of Chimney Mountain but also to an interesting view through the surrounding trees of Ship's Prow with the Chimney towering behind it.

DIRECTIONS: From NY 28 in Indian Lake, turn onto NY 30 heading south. Turn left on CR 4/Big Brook Road at 0.6 miles. Follow Big Brook Road crossing Lake Abanakee, and take a sharp right at 6.1 miles. At 7.8 miles park in the designated parking area and pay the day-use fee.

GPS Trailhead Coordinates	11 Chimney Mountain
UTM Zone (WGS 84):	18T
Easting:	0562185.1
Northing:	4837543.7
Latitude:	N 43° 41' 17.90"
Longitude:	W 74° 13' 42.25"

SCENERY: 🐾 🐾 🐾 🐾	DISTANCE: *7.5 miles*
TRAIL CONDITION: 🐾 🐾 🐾 🐾	HIKING TIME: *4–5 hours*
CHILDREN: 🐾 🐾 🐾	OUTSTANDING FEATURES: *Isolated pond,*
DIFFICULTY: 🐾	*streamside hiking*
SOLITUDE: 🐾 🐾 🐾 🐾	

Passing through this scenic notch provides hikers with excellent scenery and solitude. You follow a flat stream to a serene marsh, where Hoffman Mountain is framed in the background, and then down a fast falling brook with innumerable small cascades. The trail is fairly easy, so fast and experienced hikers will find that they can traverse the notch in half the time, but this precludes enjoying the scenery and solitude along the picturesque trail.

🏃 This point-to-point trail would be excellent in either direction but is probably easier and most enjoyable heading from south to north. Deciding which end to leave a car or where to be picked up all depends on circumstance, but it might be advisable to leave a car at the southern lot for extended trips. The southern lot is large and off the main road, while the northern end is probably easiest to give directions to. This would also be an excellent trip for the key-pass technique, where two parties start at opposite locations and exchange car keys when they pass each other, as no detours or side trips might cause them to miss each other. Directions here are given heading south to north.

The trail begins on the northwest corner of a large grassy parking area off Loch Muller Road, which has ample space for dozens of cars. A 1-mile trail to Bailey Pond, on your left, is also located at the beginning of the Hoffman Notch Trail. Continue straight ahead on the abandoned road, marked in yellow for the entire trail, through the mixed hardwood forest. The wide, open road makes

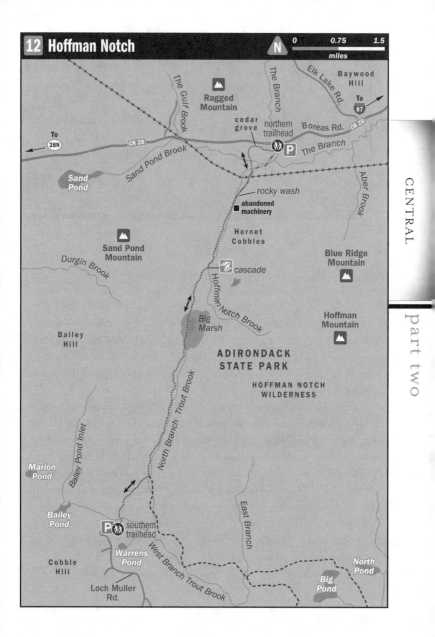

N

0   0.75   1.5
miles

Baywood
Hill

Elk Lake Rd.

The Branch

The Gulf Brook

Ragged
Mountain

cedar
grove

northern
trailhead

Boreas Rd.

To
87

CR 2B

To
28N

CR 2B

Sand Pond Brook

The Branch

Aber Brook

Sand
Pond

rocky wash

abandoned
machinery

Durgin Brook

Sand Pond
Mountain

Hornet
Cobbles

Blue Ridge
Mountain

cascade

Hoffman Notch Brook

Bailey
Hill

Big
Marsh

Hoffman
Mountain

ADIRONDACK
STATE PARK

HOFFMAN NOTCH
WILDERNESS

Bailey Pond Inlet

North Branch Trout Brook

Marion
Pond

Bailey
Pond

southern
trailhead

East Branch

Cobble
Hill

Warrens
Pond

Loch Muller
Rd.

West Branch Trout Brook

North
Pond

Big
Pond

CENTRAL

part two

for easy travel, and you will quickly come within sight of the West Branch Trout Brook approximately 0.3 miles in. The trail heads west briefly, and you descend to a recently constructed log-and-plank bridge. Like the numerous bridges near the end of the trail, the bridge has been handsomely built with substantial cribbing and stonework to bolster the crossing. Shortly after crossing the bridge, the road begins to transition into trail, but the going is still easy over the mostly rolling terrain.

You will encounter a few seasonally muddy sections before reaching the only other trail intersection at 1.3 miles. The main trail continues straight ahead following yellow disks, while the trail to the right is marked in blue and leads to another access point along Hoffman Road. If you seek an extended trip, you can add almost 6 miles by starting at Hoffman Road. The North Branch Trout Brook begins to flow on your right after you pass this intersection and accompanies you all the way to Big Marsh at the halfway point. Approximately 2 miles in, you pass an enormous erratic alongside the trail. Though many may think I am an erratic on the trail, talking into the voice recorder dangling from the front of my pack, erratics are actually large boulders that were deposited

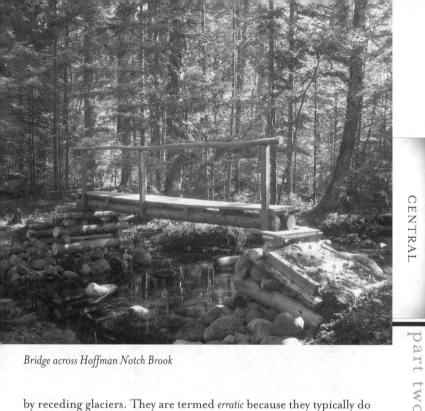

Bridge across Hoffman Notch Brook

by receding glaciers. They are termed *erratic* because they typically do not fit in with the surrounding landscape, due either to their composition or, more likely, to their location. The trail winds away from and back to the banks of the brook numerous times, and at 2.3 miles, it passes nearly through the water as it cuts its way along the mossy banks northwards. The brook flows over mostly flat terrain and consequently is very slow moving, especially so when you reach the beaver dam at 2.5 miles. Evergreens dot the banks along this section, and you will notice that the terrain is growing ever steeper on your left as you head toward the midpoint of the notch. Here, the notch is the low point between the Washburn Ridge on your left and the Texas Ridge on your right. Roughly 0.5 miles ahead, the marshland truly begins, with grassy

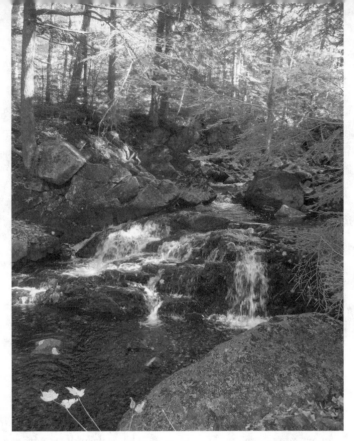

Small cascade along Hoffman Notch Brook

islands interspersed along the brook as it meanders wider near the notch's peak. The marshlands create broad, open sections in the forest, and soon Hoffman Mountain begins to loom across the scenic wetlands. At 3.5 miles the trail descends briefly to the wide, open waters of the marsh—though *lake* or *pond* would likely be a more apt description. A few skeletal trees remain in the open waters, enhancing the wild character of this remote area. Numerous vantage points for scenic photos are found all along the trail as it winds along the hemlock- and birch-lined western shore. You leave Big Marsh's shores at 4 miles, but the trail continues along flat terrain through mixed hardwoods for another 0.8 miles. A small seasonal brook joins you on your left, and shortly after it, you reach Hoffman Notch Brook. Hoffman Notch Brook tumbles in at a small cascade on your right and forms a deep pool that can be passed across a worn tree. Rock-hopping might be a better option in wet conditions, as the tree is nearly worn smooth.

The trail continues on the opposite shore under a thick canopy of hardwoods, and several wet sections turn the trail into a mire at points. At this point the brook is descending rapidly, forming innumerable cascades with a low rumbling that drowns out most other sounds of the forest. The trail parallels the brook on an elevated ridge along the eastern banks for approximately 0.3 miles before descending to the rock- and boulder-strewn brook at 5.1 miles, where you cross to the western bank. Trail markers are absent or difficult to follow in this section, but if you keep the brook in sight and look for the worn path, you can easily find your way to the crossing and the yellow trail markers. The waters are falling rapidly at this point, but the boulders are so large that it's easy to hop across the brook to the opposite shore, where the trail continues to descend on the western bank. The notch is very distinct along this portion of the trail, as you pass the several sheer rock faces of Washburn Ridge on your left and the terrain, Hornet Cobbles, grows steeper on the right. Roughly 5.8 miles in, the trail transitions into an abandoned road with built-up banks, and the hiking gets easier. At 6 miles you pass a rusted piece of abandoned track machinery on your right that reminds us of the persistent regenerative power of nature.

At 6.1 miles you reach a rocky wash where a low bridge spans Hoffman Notch Brook. This crossing marks the end of the descent, and it is mostly rolling terrain for the next 1.4 miles to the northern terminus. At 6.5 miles you pass through a clearing where power lines have cut a swath through the wilderness; shortly after, you reach another sturdy bridge that recrosses Hoffman Notch Brook. This section of the trail is a rerouting of the often-flooded north end, and a couple more excellent bridges are crossed in this flat section. The trail swings eastward through a notable stand of cedars and then intersects the old north road at 7.4 miles. The rusted front end of a classic car is found at this junction and is only a few hundred yards to the trail terminus at Boreas Road.

DIRECTIONS: *Southern Trailhead*   From US 9 in Schroon Lake, head west on County Road 24. Turn right on Potash Hill Road, 5.4 miles. At 1.1 miles turn right on Loch Muller Road. Follow Loch Muller Road 1.3 miles, and look for a gravel drive on the right. Follow the gravel drive a short way to the large grassy parking area.

Northern Trailhead   On I-87 N, take Exit 29 (CR 2-B/Boreas Road). Head west on CR 2-B/Boreas Road 5.5 miles. The parking area is a small gravel drive on the left.

GPS Trailhead Coordinates	12 Hoffman Notch
Starting Northern trailhead	
UTM Zone (WGS 84):	18T
Easting:	0593346.4
Northing:	4867412.8
Latitude:	N 43° 57' 14.12"
Longitude:	W 73° 50' 11.78"

GPS Trailhead Coordinates	12 Hoffman Notch
Ending Southern trailhead	
UTM Zone (WGS 84):	18T
Easting:	0589273.8
Northing:	4857832.1
Latitude:	N 43° 52' 5.45"
Longitude:	W 73° 53' 20.26"

13 Peaked Mountain

SCENERY: � ☆ ☆ ☆ ☆ ☆	DISTANCE: *7.2 miles*
TRAIL CONDITION: ☆ ☆ ☆ ☆	HIKING TIME: *4 hours*
CHILDREN: ☆ ☆ ☆ ☆	OUTSTANDING FEATURES: *Lakeside hiking,*
DIFFICULTY: ☆ ☆ ☆ ☆	*cascades along a stream, beaver dams and meadows,*
SOLITUDE: ☆ ☆ ☆	*isolated pond, panoramic views from a peak*

Can't choose between lakeside hiking, exploring an isolated pond, hiking beside frothy cascades, or climbing a mountain for a panoramic view? Why choose? Peaked Mountain has it all. The main trail is easy and features a variety of waterscapes, including a pristine lake, a cascading brook, and several beaver dam meadows. The last 0.8 miles along the trail are steep and difficult, but the summit has a unique perspective: At the peak, you can clearly trace your entire trip back to the shore of Thirteenth Lake.

🚶 Access to Peaked Mountain is at the north end of Thirteenth Lake, which also has car-top boat access, accessible picnic areas, and free primitive camping. Most of the vehicles in the large and spacious parking area are for camping and day use. To access the trail, walk down the main gravel drive to the trail register. The register doubles for recording day-use activities, so do not be surprised to see a lot of recorded activity. To the left is the boat launch, while access to the foot trail is down the right fork. Head toward the lake past a couple of campsites and picnic tables, and then look for the trail sign on your right near the last picnic table. Mileage given is from this point, which is a little more than 0.1 mile from the parking area.

The trail winds along the shore of Thirteenth Lake, weaving through paper birches and other hardwoods. Beaver activity is evident everywhere, from chewed stumps and recently felled trees across the path to several lodges that are within feet of the trail. The trail is relatively flat with a few dips and hills that follow the contours of the lake. You will encounter a couple of designated

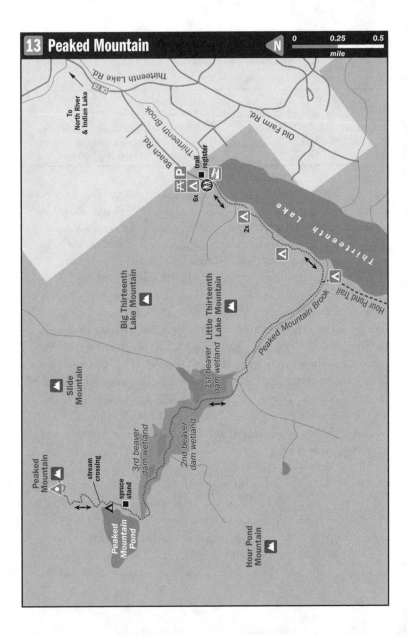

N

0	0.25	0.5
mile		

To
North River
& Indian Lake

Thirteenth Lake Rd.

CR 78

Beach Rd.

Thirteenth Brook

Old Farm Rd.

trail
register

P

6x

2x

Thirteenth Lake

Big Thirteenth
Lake Mountain

Little Thirteenth
Lake Mountain

1st beaver
dam wetland

Peaked Mountain Brook

Hour Pond Trail

Slide
Mountain

3rd beaver
dam wetland

2nd beaver
dam wetland

Peaked
Mountain

stream
crossing

spruce
stand

Peaked
Mountain
Pond

Hour Pond
Mountain

primitive campsites along the trail as well, so be aware that you may be walking through or near someone's site. The shores of Thirteenth Lake are undeveloped and pristine. Though not common, motorboaters are occasionally heard, which is odd because the lake is nestled in the middle of a wilderness area. (Wilderness Area land-use plans typically preclude the use of motorized boats; hopefully the state will enforce this standard in the future.) Typically, the lake will be dotted with canoeists and kayakers, and in fact, many of these boaters paddle to where the trail diverges from the lake, around 0.8 miles on the right.

This junction occurs where Peaked Mountain Brook empties into Thirteenth Lake. Shortly after you begin following the brook uphill, you encounter a trail sign indicating Hour Pond to your left. However, to reach Peaked Mountain and its pond, continue uphill alongside the brook. You will be following Peaked Mountain Brook through numerous transformations all the way to the pond and the foot of the mountain. Innumerable small falls and cascades characterize the brook until you cross it upstream, at 1.5 miles, and provide an interesting contrast to the flat and quiet waters of the lake behind

CENTRAL

part two

you. You will have to rock-hop across the brook to a tiny island and then again to the opposite bank.

The trail levels off after crossing the brook. Shortly after, you will notice a clearing to your right. This clearing is a result of the first dammed section of the brook. From the trail, hemlocks frame the grassy wetland and an outstanding view of Slide Mountain. Farther along, the trail winds closer to the wetland, and looking east, you will see Big Thirteenth Lake Mountain. This is the first of three distinct beaver-dammed sections along the brook, but with all the evident beaver activity, the landscape could easily change from year to year. It is tempting to think that one of these dammed sections is Peaked Mountain Pond and that one of the mountains is Peaked Mountain. However, the pond is a broader expanse of still water, and Peaked Mountain has exposed sheer faces with less tree cover.

After looking across the wetland at Big Thirteenth Lake Mountain, you will pass very close to a large beaver dam at 1.9 miles. Shortly after, you recross the brook and head back into the woods briefly before another wetland opens up to your left. A couple of rocks along the trail's edge provide a good vantage point of the dammed wetland, which surrounds a tiny cedar-dotted island. The trail hugs the eastern edge of this wetland and then recrosses Peaked Mountain Brook at the northern edge of the wetland. The crossing is little more than a step across the brook, where it passes between two broad rocks, and you are roughly two-thirds of the way to the pond. The third and final major dammed section gives you the first real glimpse of Peaked Mountain's large exposed face. A lot more large dead trees are in this section, with the additional distinction of large boulders strewn about.

After a short section of walking through dense woods, you climb a small hill to discover Peaked Mountain Pond straight ahead at 3 miles. At this point, paths lead off to your left, and the trail is to your right. A fallen tree makes this a convenient spot to sit next to the pond. However, a nice place to rest is also a little farther up the trail in a small area of spruces. The trail so far has been fairly easy and

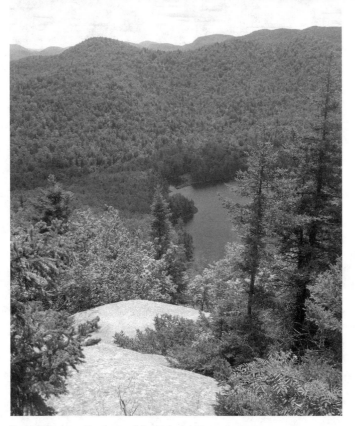

Peaked Mountain Pond viewed from a lookout near the peak

accessible to most hikers. However, the climb to the summit is much steeper and requires a lot more effort. It is certainly worth the ascent, so take time to rest and enjoy the view of the beautiful pond.

The trail up the mountain passes through the stand of spruces previously mentioned and past a fork in the trail, which indicates a designated camping area to the left. The trail climbs slightly, among beeches and maples, and then descends to a stream crossing with

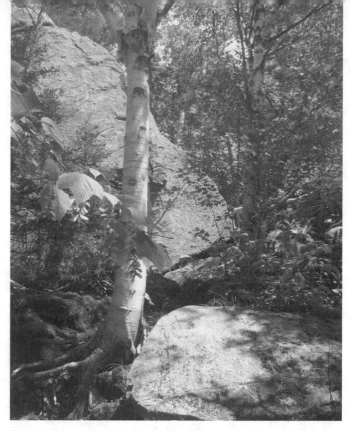

Exposed portions of ledge along the climb to Peaked Mountain

views of the pond to your left. Climbing begins immediately after you cross the stream. This section is steep with large exposed rocks, and the forest is almost entirely paper birches. Blown-down birches often cover the trail, making spotting the actual trail and finding the best footing difficult at times. However, red disks mark the trail, and alternate paths around the blowdown are evident. After the first steep section, the grade eases a bit through a section where sheer rock is on your left and a rock hump is to your right. The trail swings to your left, just past a massive boulder, and becomes steep again. Climbing is steady until just before the top, and there are several tricky spots, so take your time and make room for other hikers as they pass. When evergreens dominate the forest, you'll know that you are close to the summit. A large open portion of bedrock provides excellent views down onto the pond, but the best part is at the true summit. After a brief foray back into the evergreens, you are once again out in the open. Sprawling out beneath you is your entire trip from where you left Thirteenth Lake. Peaked Mountain Pond and the beaver-dammed sections are obvious, as is the path the brook has cut into the landscape. In the height of summer, dragonflies perform aerial acrobatics for your viewing pleasure, and the bedrock provides a great spot to sit and look out at the beautiful vista.

DIRECTIONS: Heading west along NY 28, turn right onto County Road 78/Thirteenth Lake Road, 12.1 miles past the intersection of NY 28 and NY 30 in Indian Lake Village. Bear right onto Beach Road at 3.3 miles. End at the large parking area at 0.7 miles.

GPS Trailhead Coordinates	13 Peaked Mountain
UTM Zone (WGS 84):	18T
Easting:	0570958.7
Northing:	4840838.4
Latitude:	N 43° 43' 1.85"
Longitude:	W 74° 07' 8.83"

CENTRAL

part two

14 Shanty Brook

SCENERY: ✿ ✿ ✿ ✿	DISTANCE: *7.6 miles*
TRAIL CONDITION: ✿ ✿	HIKING TIME: *4–5 hours*
CHILDREN: ✿ ✿ ✿	OUTSTANDING FEATURES: *Waterfall,*
DIFFICULTY: ✿ ✿	*swimming hole, remote pond*
SOLITUDE: ✿ ✿ ✿ ✿	

Although not difficult, this unmarked trail varies from a narrow footpath to an out-right bushwhack, so unseasoned hikers should be prepared before undertaking this adventure. One of the more notable preparations is to expect to have wet feet. There is almost no getting around this, so plan accordingly, and you will be able to enjoy the beautiful waterfall, swimming hole, and remote pond.

👫 Most of the parking areas along NY 8 are unmarked, so finding the right one can be tricky. Fortunately, paying attention to your odometer readings and your GPS should steer you in the right direction. The parking area for Shanty Brook is distinct because it is on the south side of the road and is the only one that is U-shaped; most are large lots or gravel pulloffs right next to the road. The trail is unmarked, and although portions are well worn, this hike definitely counts as a bushwhack. You have to wade across the East Branch of the Sacandaga River, so either bring water shoes or plan to hike in wet boots. Additionally, the rocks in the river are slippery, so a change of clothes in a dry sack will be appreciated should the crossing not go according to plan.

To reach the river crossing, head northeast along NY 8 a few hundred feet to where a short dirt road provides access to a designated campsite along the river. A steep drop-off leads down to the East Branch of the Sacandaga River on the left-hand side of the road. Across the river, you will see where Shanty Brook meets the river, and you should start looking for a good crossing point. The trail is on the

Stockholm
Brook

Black
Mountain

small
island

CENTRAL

informal
campsite

Shanty Brook

beaver
dam

Mud
Ponds

**ADIRONDACK
STATE PARK**

SIAMESE POND
WILDERNESS

part two

Blue Hills

waterfall

Shanty Brook

8

old
wooden stand

P   To
     Wells

E. Branch
Sacandaga River

west side of the brook, and I found that an easy way down to the river is about midway down the road, where an old wooden stand provides access to a cable crossing. The cable crossing is washed away, but the stand remains a good landmark. This is less than 100 feet downriver from the confluence of the brook and river. On the opposite shore, you can see where the vegetation has been beaten down where the cable used to be connected. Carefully wade across the river, or rock-hop if the season has been dry enough; do not count on keeping your feet dry.

On the opposite shore, a well-worn path leads to the western shore of the brook. The trail parallels the brook and crosses several muddy sections as you begin a gentle climb. A little less than 0.8 miles in, you will see a path to your right and notice that the rumble of the brook has gotten louder. Follow the path to the right to reach the top of the waterfall. The falls plunge 12 feet, though they seem taller, into a deep pool that is enclosed within the steep banks of the brook. To reach the base of the waterfall and the swimming hole, jump across the brook to the opposite shore and scramble down the banks over roots and rocks to the base of the falls. The pool at the base of the falls is not large but is deep enough to swim in, and you

Shanty Brook seen above the falls

can swim right into the falls. A little upstream on the east shore is a designated campsite that would be ideal for a short overnight trip.

Back along the main trail, the path climbs a bit more but quickly levels off for essentially the rest of the trip. A quarter mile from the falls, the trail veers away from the brook but then turns briefly eastward and crosses the brook 0.8 miles from the falls, 1.5 miles from the start. You will pass an open area and beaver dam along the brook at approximately 2.3 miles. This is the first of two open areas along the brook that provide views of the surrounding hills. At the second open area, 2.6 miles, the trail seems to abruptly terminate in a sandy wash. The meadow lies straight before you, rather than to your left as it was previously. This is where you need to recross the brook to reach

Shanty Brook Falls

Mud Ponds. The path on the opposite shore is hard to discern in the summer growth and flooded-out areas, but as long as you keep the brook on your right, you will eventually find a well-worn section of the path. I found that following a small seasonal channel between an evergreen-dotted island on your right and the surrounding hillside to your left, you can more easily work your way northward to the more distinct portions of the path.

The trail from this point on is not traveled as heavily, and blow-down and washouts make navigating a little more difficult. Hikers who are not familiar with basic navigation, lack a compass and map or a good sense of direction, or are uncomfortable with unmarked trails would probably be better served returning before the crossing rather than finishing the hike to Mud Ponds. Additionally, gaiters provide a welcome reprieve from the leg lashings of brambles and fallen trees that encroach on the trail.

A third of a mile from the recrossing, 3 miles from the start, the trail swings westward as you follow Shanty Brook, now on your right, toward Mud Ponds. The brook now flows over mostly level ground and is much more placid than before. At 3.2 miles, you reach what appears to be the eastern tip of Mud Ponds but is only a widening of the brook due to beaver activity. The actual eastern tip is at 3.6 miles. The path weaves its way along the southern shore of the pond through thick overgrowth and wet sections. At 3.7 miles, you pass a grassy channel that connects the two main ponds and soon reach a small hill that lies between the ponds. Atop this hill is an informal campsite with benches and a fire pit, which, for all intents and purposes, marks the end of the bushwhack. Farther on are more paths, but they soon end in impassable brambles or mires.

DIRECTIONS: From the intersection of NY 30 and NY 8 in Wells, follow NY 8 east 8.9 miles. The parking area is on your left in the shape of a U.

From the intersection of NY 28 and NY 8 in Wevertown, follow NY 8 west 14.5 miles. The parking area is on your right and is in the shape of a U.

GPS Parking Area Coordinates	14 Shanty Brook
UTM Zone (WGS 84):	18T
Easting:	0569337.4
Northing:	4820419.1
Latitude:	N 43° 32' 7.58"
Longitude:	W 74° 08' 30.69"

GPS Trailhead Coordinates	14 Shanty Brook
UTM Zone (WGS 84):	18T
Easting:	0569409.1
Northing:	4820623.5
Latitude:	N 43° 32' 14.18"
Longitude:	W 74° 08' 27.40"

SCENERY: ✿ ✿ ✿ ✿	DISTANCE: *2.4 miles round-trip either route*
TRAIL CONDITION: ✿ ✿ ✿	HIKING TIME: *1–2 hours*
CHILDREN: ✿ ✿	OUTSTANDING FEATURES: *Waterfall,*
DIFFICULTY: ✿ ✿	*swimming hole, scenic river gorge*
SOLITUDE: ✿ ✿ ✿ ✿	

The East Branch of the Sacandaga River has a spectacular gorge with a serene waterfall and swimming hole that you can reach in two different ways. The most direct and clearest route is to follow the southern footpath to Square Falls. The most scenic and adventurous route is to ford the river and then bushwhack along the northern banks. Neither route is very long, and the two are easily combined if you choose to ford the river twice.

🚶🚶 There are no trail signs or indications of the trailhead either in the expansive parking area or from NY 8, so pay attention to your odometer, as numerous unmarked parking areas are along NY 8. Additionally, there is no trail register, and the trail is not marked, but if you pay attention to the directions below, the paths are fairly easy to find and follow. The trail begins on the northeastern edge of the parking area along an old road. The abandoned dirt road descends from the main road into the forest in a general northwesterly direction. Approximately 0.1 mile down, you reach the end of the road and a turnaround on your left. Large boulders on your right barricade the remaining trail from vehicular travel. Wind your way down the trail to the small stream crossing shortly ahead. Once across the stream, you must decide which route you will choose to explore the gorge. The path along the southern edge is hard to make out amid the debris of seasonal flooding but is easily distinguished by climbing the tiny hill directly to your right. The northern bushwhack is accessed by continuing straight ahead and then heading toward the river along numerous footpaths. Both options, described separately

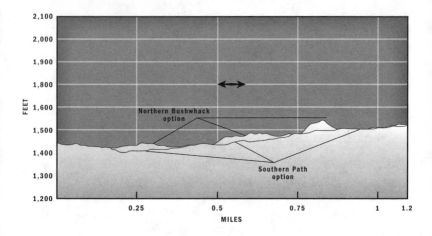

below, terminate at Square Falls, where you can easily ford the river if you wish to combine the trips. If you choose to take the southern path and return along the northern edge, then you should scope out the condition of the river now before continuing. There are two reasons to do so: First, you will need to recognize where to recross the river; second, you will need to determine whether the river is shallow enough to rock-hop or if wading in the strong current will be necessary. Upriver, several narrow areas make crossing easier.

Northern Bushwhack

Upon reaching the banks of the East Branch of the Sacandaga River, you will face the decision of where to cross. Only hikers who are nimble and willing to wade should attempt the crossing. Downriver, a double cable was once strung to assist hikers in crossing during high water, but only a single cable remains. Clearly, the remaining cable is the upper one, and to use it you would have to shimmy hand over hand with legs locked behind you across dozens of feet and high above the water. Rock-hopping is a better choice and might get you across (or, as I found, most of the way across) with short sections remaining

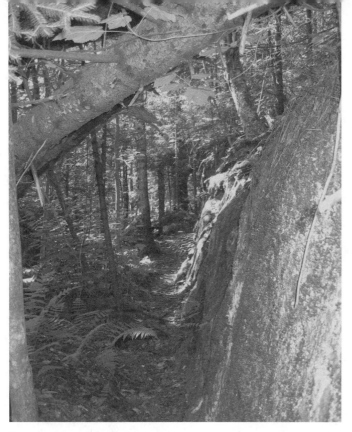

Eight-foot ledge beside the trail

to be waded. Despite appearing relatively flat, the current is strong, and the round rocks that line the riverbed are slick with slime, so be mindful of your footing. Now that the caveats have been established, let us recognize that in summer, wading across the river can be quite fun and refreshing. Besides, you are headed to a swimming hole. I found an excellent and easily recognizable section to cross upriver where two large boulders sit on the southern bank.

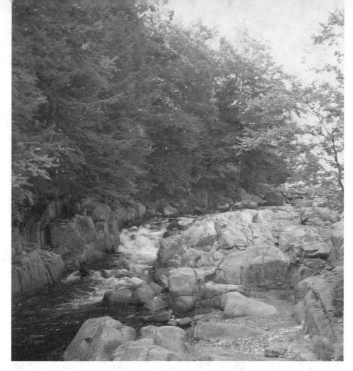

Small cascade along the river

Once on the opposite bank, the path is not readily clear, but rest assured that you will find it if you head upriver close to the rocky banks. Hemlock saplings crowd the banks, while mature trees shade the north side of the river. The informal path on this side of the river is distinct in some areas and disappears among the dense saplings and fallen trees in others, but if you keep the river within sight on your right, you will find your way to the falls. Roughly 0.3 miles into the hike, the gorge begins with a small cascade among the boulder-strewn banks. As you hike, you will notice that the bank on the southern side is nearly vertical; in sections it ranges from 50–100 feet high, and with the frothy water churning beneath, the scenery has a distinctly wild and rugged character. Approximately 0.5 miles into the hike, the steep riverbanks draw close together with a nearly 20-foot drop to the river. A double cable strung between large eastern white pines on the opposing banks provides another crossing over a deep pool. I don't recommend this crossing except for experienced hikers who have a means to tie off and are in the company of other hikers. Above the pool, the river contracts to a narrow flume through which it spurts out a torrent of foam. You will pass several other small cascades on your way upriver, all of which may seem like Square Falls. However, you won't reach Square Falls until you have hiked 1.2 miles; you can distinguish it from the other cascades because it forms a six- to eight-foot cascade across the entire river. Additionally, a wide pool lies at its base, while a broad, tabular portion of bedrock forms its top.

SOUTHERN PATH

Following the southern path is by far the easiest, safest, and fastest approach to the falls. If it were not for the dramatic scenery offered along the northern bushwhack and the lack of scenery on this bank, I would recommend this route to all hikers. Once on this well-trodden path, it is hard to lose. For the most part, the path winds atop the gorge cliffs, so views of the river and the dramatic walls are obscured by dense foliage below, but the torrent of water can be heard most of the way. Roughly 0.3 miles in, you arrive at the cascade at the end of the gorge, where an old fire pit is situated close to the riverbank. A tenth of a mile ahead, you pass the double-cable crossing described above. At 0.6 miles, the trail climbs very steeply away from the banks, and you walk high above the river for 0.3 miles before winding your way back down to the river. You have passed the gorge portion of the hike, but the falls and swimming hole await you 0.3 miles ahead. The river is visible along this last portion of the trail and makes for some beautiful scenery, but this route has nowhere near the dramatic contrasts of the northern bushwhack.

DIRECTIONS: From the intersection of NY 30 and NY 8 in Wells, travel east on NY 8. The parking area is 11.7 miles ahead on your left.

From the intersection of NY 28 and NY 8 in Wevertown, head west on NY 8. The parking area is 11.7 miles ahead on your right.

GPS Trailhead Coordinates	15 West Branch Sacandaga Gorge
UTM Zone (WGS 84):	18T
Easting:	0571637.0
Northing:	4824443.4
Latitude:	N 43° 34' 10.24"
Longitude:	W 74° 06' 46.34"

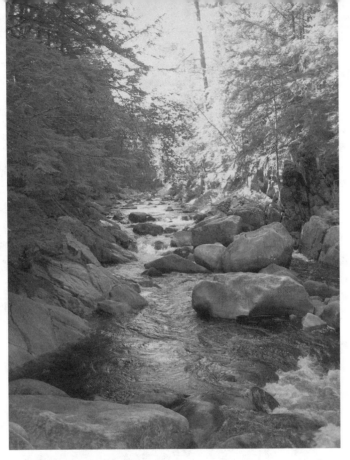

The East Branch of the Sacandaga River

Eastern Hikes (16–20)

N

0   2.5   5
miles

74

16 17

Schroon Lake

Pharaoh
Mountain

87

Schroon Lake

Hague

8

Trout Brook

Pottersville

9

Brant Lake

ADIRONDACK
STATE PARK

9N

Schroon River

8

87

Panther
Mountain

20

The Glen

9

Cat
Mountain

Erebus
Mountain

28

9N

18

19

Hudson River

Schroon River

Lake George

Warrensburg

87

3

PART THREE
Eastern Hikes

SCENERY: ✿ ✿ ✿ ✿	DISTANCE: 5.8–9.4 miles
TRAIL CONDITION: ✿ ✿ ✿ ✿ ✿	HIKING TIME: 4–6 hours
CHILDREN: ✿ ✿ ✿	OUTSTANDING FEATURES: Spectacular views,
DIFFICULTY: ✿ ✿ ✿	scenic marsh
SOLITUDE: ✿ ✿ ✿	

An excellent peak in the eastern section of the Adirondacks, Pharaoh Mountain is an exceptional destination in itself or as a side trip in the heart of the Pharaoh Lake Wilderness. Accessibility along the rough and partially flooded Crane Pond Road will determine the total length of the hike and can extend it by 3.8 miles round-trip.

👣 Though Crane Pond Road is officially closed at the end of the pavement, where a small parking area has been established, locals and others accessing Crane Pond and Pharaoh Lake Wilderness routinely use it. The road was barricaded in the 1980s, but local residents removed the barricade the following spring. When Earth First! tried to erect a new barrier, a conflict arose that involved a pugilistic encounter between a local politician and an Earth First! representative. The whole encounter was caught on camera and eventually made it to the national news. At present, there are no barriers, and the road is left open and used by hikers, anglers, boaters, and campers alike. However, the road is not maintained and is very rough. You need a high-clearance, four-wheel-drive vehicle if you wish to drive the remaining 1.9 miles to the Crane Pond parking area.

The rough road winds through a dense forest and is pleasant for walking or driving. Keep an eye out for spots to pull off the main road, as there are few and they usually can accommodate only one vehicle. Approximately 1.6 miles in, the road descends to a flooded section, which varies in depth and length, depending on recent rain and the season. It is almost always flooded, so do not count on being

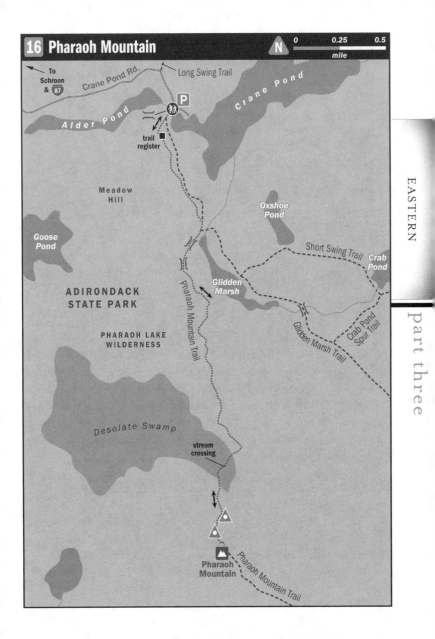

N

0   0.25   0.5
mile

To
Schroon
& 87

Crane Pond Rd.

Long Swing Trail

Crane Pond

P

Alder Pond

trail register

Meadow Hill

Oxshoe Pond

Short Swing Trail

Crab Pond

Goose Pond

ADIRONDACK
STATE PARK

Glidden Marsh

Pharaoh Mountain Trail

PHARAOH LAKE
WILDERNESS

Glidden Marsh Trail

Crab Pond Spur Trail

Desolate Swamp

stream crossing

Pharaoh Mountain

Pharaoh Mountain Trail

able to drive farther. However, the base is solid cobbles and passable during low water conditions, as long as you do not stop or drive too fast. If it is not passable or you are apprehensive about crossing, find parking either on the side of the road nearby or back at the initial lot, and use the bypass trail to the north the flooded section. Past the flooded section, the road continues to wind through the forest, passing Long Swing Trail at 1.7 miles and eventually reaching the first of two grassy parking areas. If you thought one would have to be crazy to ford the flooded section, you will be surprised to find several vehicles that made the crossing. Whether you are driving or hiking, it is 1.9 miles from the initial parking area. Trail description and mileage will be given from this point.

Proceed east to the boat launch and second parking area, and then head south past a downed pine tree and a trail sign on your right. A wide bridge crosses the outlet of Crane Pond, which is on your left, as it flows into Alder Pond on your right. The trail, marked by red disks, uses primarily old access roads, so it is broad and free of obstructions. Additionally, there are very few muddy areas, so this trail is one of the few in the Adirondacks that are in exceptional

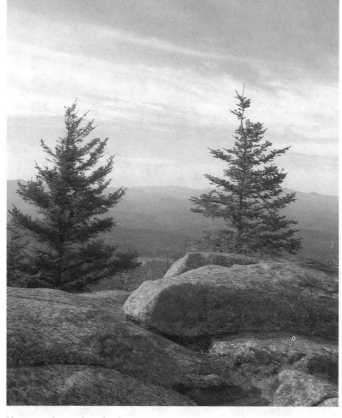

View atop the northern knob

condition. The wide trail climbs gently as it winds through a mostly hemlock forest for a little less than 0.3 miles to the trail register. It continues over level terrain for another 0.5 miles under the canopy of towering hemlocks and eastern white pines to a fork in the trail. This intersection, 0.7 miles from Crane Pond, is situated on the northern tip of Glidden Marsh. Looming straight ahead over the marsh's placid water is Pharaoh Mountain. To the right is the direct approach to the summit, as well as a route to Pharaoh Lake, while on

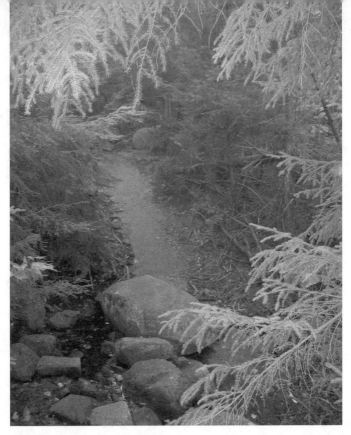

Portion of the trail on the way to the summit

the left is another route to Pharaoh Lake via Glidden Marsh. If you
desire a longer trip, descend from the summit to Pharaoh Lake, skirt
the lakeshore on the northern trail (not shown on most maps), and
then head back along Glidden Marsh Trail for a circuit of 7.3 miles.
For a description of the return leg along Glidden Marsh, see the
Pharaoh Lake overnight section on page 131.

Bear right at the fork in the trail and proceed along the western
shore of Glidden Marsh. You will cross a couple of log bridges as you

navigate the next 0.3 miles of level terrain. At 1 mile, the climb to the summit begins. As you ascend, the forest transitions from the towering evergreens to a mostly hardwood forest. The mixture features oak and cherry trees at first, and then gives way to predominately maple and beech. At 1.7 miles, you reach a fork with an overgrown abandoned road on the left, but the trail continues on your right. The easy hiking along old roads gives way to rougher hiking as you pick your way along exposed bedrock and through the rocks and cobbles that dominate the trail. Approximately 2 miles in, the canopy height begins to diminish, and the forest transitions back to evergreens, though the composition is now stunted firs dotted with birches.

At 2.3 miles, you will have to rock-hop across a stream, and the climbing becomes much steeper. Over the next 0.5 miles, the trees become stunted, and the trail, flanked by alpine mosses, crosses over exposed portions of bedrock. As you approach the summit, several exposed ledges are either on the trail or mere feet to your right, with amazing views to the north and west. I suggest taking some time to admire the views to the north, as the panorama at the summit is mostly to the west and south. At the summit, the trail passes through a shallow cleft that bisects what are essentially the two summits of Pharaoh Mountain. The northern knob is to your left and has exceptional views to the west, especially of Schroon Lake. Footpaths meander about the northern knob, where a couple of informal campsites are interspersed among the windswept firs. Follow the main path a very short distance farther south to find the footpath that leads to the southern knob. From the exposed portions of bedrock on this knob are excellent views down on Pharaoh Lake.

Note: The Pharaoh Lake overnight trail begins at the end of this trail.

DIRECTIONS: From the intersection of US 9 and NY 73/NY 74, near Exit 28 on I-87 N, head south on US 9. Turn left onto Alder Meadow Road at 0.6 miles. Follow Alder Meadow Road 2.1 miles, and bear left onto Crane Pond Road. The parking lot is on the left where the pavement ends, and Crane Pond Road turns into an unmaintained road at 1.4 miles.

GPS Parking Area Coordinates	16 Pharaoh Mountain
UTM Zone (WGS 84):	18T
Easting:	0605376.4
Northing:	4857052.5
Latitude:	N 43° 51' 32.55"
Longitude:	W 73° 41' 19.54"
GPS Trailhead Coordinates	16 Pharaoh Mountain
UTM Zone (WGS 84):	18T
Easting:	0607494.3
Northing:	4856227.2
Latitude:	N 43° 51' 4.70"
Longitude:	W 73° 39' 45.29"

17 Pharaoh Lake

SCENERY: ✴ ✴ ✴ ✴	DISTANCE: *14.4 miles*
TRAIL CONDITION: ✴ ✴ ✴ ✴	HIKING TIME: *Overnight*
CHILDREN: ✴ ✴	OUTSTANDING FEATURES: *Exceptional lake-*
DIFFICULTY: ✴ ✴ ✴	*side camping, waterfall*
SOLITUDE: ✴ ✴ ✴	

The lean-tos and designated campsites along the shores of Pharaoh Lake are some of the best in the Adirondacks. The sheer number of sites in this virtual wilderness camp-ground means that you will likely find a spot even on busy holiday weekends. If you crave solitude, choose an off-peak weekend or shy away from the lean-tos and pick a remote tent site. The designated sites and lean-tos are nearly all next to the shore with excellent views, and it's clear why they are popular.

🚶🚶 Numerous trails lead to Pharaoh Lake, but the description provided here is from the end of Pharaoh Mountain Trail described on page 124. Bear in mind that parking for the Pharaoh Mountain trailhead is either at the designated parking area at the end of the pavement on Crane Pond Road or at the end of the unmaintained portion, which is technically closed and requires fording a stream. Consequently, total mileage will depend on where you park. See the Pharaoh Mountain Trail description for details.

From the end of Pharaoh Mountain Trail, descend the southern slope following the red trail markers, 2.9 miles from Crane Pond. Shortly after leaving the summit, you must climb down a vertical portion of exposed ledge that is several feet high and requires the use of both hands. Footholds are available in a small cleft next to the adjoining sheer rock face on your right. The descent is steeper than the climb to the summit, and the forest quickly transforms from alpine evergreens and birches to a dense maple-beech forest. At 4.3 miles, a sheer cliff looms to your right and indicates that you

N

| 0 | 0.5 | 1 |

mile

To Schroon & 87

Short Swing Trail

Crane Pond Rd.

Long Swing Trail

P

Alder Pond

Crane Pond

trail register

Meadow Hill

Burge Pond

Antwine Hill

Pine Hill

Honey Pond

Rock Pond Brook

Rock Pond to Lilypad Pond Trail

Lilypad Pond

Peaked Hill

Goose Pond

Oxshoe Pond

Horseshoe Pond

Glidden Marsh

Short Swing Trail

Crab Pond

Short Swing Trail

Treadway Mountain

Treadway Mountain Trail

Crab Pond Spur Trail

Glidden Marsh Trail

Desolate Swamp

ADIRONDACK STATE PARK

Devils Washdish

Grizzle Ocean Trail

Pharaoh Mountain

Pharaoh Mountain Trail

PHARAOH LAKE WILDERNESS

lean-to

Split Rock Bay

Winter Green Point Trail

waterfall

Pharaoh Lake

lean-to

Wolf Pond

Sucker Brook Trail

Watch Rocks lean-to

Desolate Brook

Pharaoh Lake Brook

Whortleberry Pond Trail

Springhill Pond from West Trail

are nearing the lakeshore. Soon after, you traverse a wet section
across planks laid lengthwise. By now, you can catch masked glimpses
of the lake through the thick beech saplings. At 4.5 miles, you reach
the intersection with the north lakeside trail. From here, you can
circle the lake in either direction. Counterclockwise, to your right,
is the fastest and most direct approach to the majority of the lean-tos.
On the other hand, heading clockwise brings you to some of the best
campsites, as well as Split Rock Bay and the final return route via
Glidden Marsh. This trail is not shown on most maps of the area.
The description and mileage here will be in the clockwise direction.

Turn left and follow the west shore trail, marked with blue disks,
toward Split Rock Bay. This portion of the trail is roughly 0.7 miles
long and follows the shoreline very closely. It also features three
excellent designated camping areas. The first of these is just off the
trail at 4.7 miles. A fire pit has been placed along an exposed portion
of ledge within feet of the lake, and a long, rocky peninsula makes a
superb spot to admire the view. A little less than 0.3 miles ahead, you
will pass a yellow DEC designated camping disk with an arrow. These
arrow disks indicate that a designated site is nearby. Usually these

sites are farther off the trail and can be easily located by following the arrows. On occasion, disks will be missing or the indicated direction of the arrow may lead you astray, so use the disks as a means to zero in on the spot rather than as absolute markers. In this case, wander out along the southern edge of the peninsula, just below an elevated ridge, and you will find the picturesque site. Surrounded by tall pines and small blueberry bushes, it sits high on the elevated peninsula and offers commanding views of the lake.

Back along the loop, the trail dips down and follows a cattail-filled bay briefly before reaching another designated camping disk at 5 miles. To reach this site, head east onto another small peninsula, where you will find a site very similar to the last one near the peninsula's tip. The intersection with Glidden Marsh Trail back to Crane Pond is at 5.1 miles.

Shortly after the intersection, the trail, now marked in yellow, winds along another bay with large boulders sticking up in the middle. This is Split Rock Bay, and while the rocks do look split from this shore, their appearance from the opposite shore is more dramatic. From the opposing shore, the split rocks appear to be a pair of obelisks with an eerie and unnatural quality. On your way to the opposite shore, you will pass an abandoned fiberglass boat, which, had you come in the other direction, would not seem unusual. At 5.7 miles, you reach lean-to 4 (also known as Split Rock Bay lean-to), which is within a couple dozen feet of the shore and has an open view south out onto the lake.

It's likely that you will see a boat pulled up on the shore nearby, and the mystery of the abandoned boat will start to resolve itself. In fact, all the lean-tos around the lake have some sort of boat, usually a canoe or small rowboat, located nearby. Improvised paddles are typically found nearby as well, but they are, in some cases, little more than flat logs. If you have the foresight to pack an ultralight paddle, you could easily become the most popular guest at the lake.

The trail swings northeast at the lean-to and heads into a thick hemlock forest. This area is heavily shaded and has few saplings, so the views into the surrounding forest are expansive. Dotted with mossy wet areas, this brief foray into a hemlock swamp is a pleasant change of pace from the standard hardwoods, but the trail delves back into mixed hardwoods after 0.4 miles. At 6.4 miles, you reach another intersection. To your right is a side trip to Winter Green Point, marked with red disks, while straight ahead is the continuation of the lakeside trail. The less than 0.3-mile side trip to the rocky point is definitely worthwhile and provides excellent views of the lake as well as Pharaoh Mountain.

Back on the trail, you quickly reach another fork; to the left are Grizzly Ocean and Putnam Pond Campground, 5.8 miles away, while the lakeside trail continues straight ahead. Roughly 0.3 miles ahead, you reach a wide stream crossing where the log cribbing is all that remains of an old bridge. You can easily rock-hop across, but you might want to bushwhack a short distance upstream to where a tiny waterfall splashes into a deep boulder-dammed pool. The trail winds up and down a few hillocks through a mixed pine forest before reaching another intersection at 6.7 miles. Lean-to 3 is off to your right, while the east shore trail continues ahead. The lean-to sits on an elevated cliff along the lake and offers outstanding views. The ledge has several wide step-downs before it finally drops to the lakeshore, all of which make excellent spots to dally.

The trail continues southwesterly among the mixed pines for a while, and you reach another designated campsite at 7.1 miles. The site is just off the trail but is quite close to the lake and is a good spot for anyone wishing to avoid the crowds that congregate at lean-tos. From this point on, many portions of the east shore trail hug the shoreline, and views of Pharaoh Mountain are superb. An abundance of highbush blueberries crowds the trail along the exposed portions of lichen-covered ledge that form the shoreline and much of the trail. At 7.4 miles, you cross a plank bridge to a small peninsula and pass an informal campsite that sees regular use. A quarter mile later you pass a designated campsite that has exceptional views of Pharaoh Mountain across the lake.

You reach another major intersection at 8 miles. To the left and marked in red are Springhill Pond, 4.5 miles, and New Hague Road, 8.3 miles, while the east shore trail continues straight ahead, still marked in yellow. Shortly ahead, you reach lean-to 2. This is the largest of the lean-tos, double the capacity of the others, and has a pleasant grassy field that slopes down to the lake in front of it. The view is less desirable than in other locations but seems very popular nonetheless. The trail toward the outlet and lean-to 1 is an old road that passes through a tall hemlock and pine forest. The wide road is free of obstructions and allows deep views into the surrounding forest. As you come down a slight hill, you see the side of lean-to 1. Close to the shore, it has beautiful views of the north shore and, like the rest of the lean-tos, has a watercraft stowed nearby.

The wide road continues south to the outlet of the lake, but you have to pass through a long mire before the canopy opens up at the grassy southern tip of the lake, 8.8 miles. The trail, now marked with red disks, heads north along the lakeshore, and you quickly reach another yellow camping disk with an arrow indicating a site nearby. The site lies atop the small knoll to your right. Though it's high above the water, views of the lake are shielded by a rise in the hill and the saplings that line the hill. Nonetheless, it is a fine site and ideal for those seeking privacy and a sheltered setting. A little more than 0.3 miles from the outlet, you reach a fork in the trail; veer left to follow the trail, or head right following yellow disks to lean-to 6. Though it is situated more than 100 yards from the lakeshore, it has excellent views, and the deep evergreen forest that shades the site makes it feel uniquely isolated.

The trail continues north, winding through hemlock groves along the lakeshore and up into deciduous hilltops. At 9.5 miles, you pass another designated site, which is situated on the forest side of the trail. This is probably the least desirable of the sites but would make a good stopping point if the lean-tos are full and night is coming on. At 9.7 miles, you reach yet another fork in the trail. To your left is the main trail, while straight ahead is lean-to 5 (also known as Watch Rocks lean-to). The lean-to trail is marked in yellow and closely follows the shoreline. Located near the tip of the peninsula, it has views in all directions, the most exceptional being at the point itself.

The main trail, rougher here than in other sections, climbs slightly and weaves its way mostly through a thick hardwood forest. The lake is no longer visible, and there is very little of note until you return to the intersection with Pharaoh Mountain Trail, 10.5 miles. Continue until you reach the intersection with Glidden Marsh Trail, 11.1 miles. Emblazoned with yellow disks, Glidden Marsh Trail climbs away from the lake immediately. The rocky climb is through mostly deciduous forest, and there are noticeably more ash trees along the slope than elsewhere along the hike. After roughly 0.3 miles, the trail levels off as you begin to pass a broad wetland on your right. The wetland, the result of beaver activity, becomes quite broad, and the trail often passes through its muddy edges for the next mile. The trail leaves the marshy section and reenters the forest as you begin a 0.3-mile descent to another fork in the trail. Straight ahead and marked in yellow is Crane Pond, while off to the right is Crab Pond Spur Trail that passes Crab and Horseshoe ponds.

Shortly after this intersection at 12.7 miles, a log bridge spans a feeder stream of Glidden Marsh, and you reach the eastern shore of the marsh soon after. The trail closely follows the broad, grassy marshland, where you can see several beaver lodges in the center of the deeper water. At 13.3 miles, you come to the intersection with Short Swing Trail, which passes Oxshoe Pond, on your right. The main trail, Glidden Marsh Trail, and Short Swing Trail are marked with blue disks. You lose sight of Glidden Marsh as you pass on the eastern side of a small hill that flanks the marsh. Another marsh down to your right is a dammed stream that feeds Crane Pond before the trail turns west. The trail crosses a log bridge and then climbs a rocky hill before descending to the intersection with Pharaoh Mountain Trail. Heading north on the old abandoned road, the mileage is

EASTERN

part three

137

as follows: less than 0.5 miles to the trail register, 0.7 miles to the Crane Pond parking area, and 2.6 miles to the designated parking area. This section of the trail is marked in red disks and is easy to follow, but for a more thorough description, read the Pharaoh Mountain Trail section.

DIRECTIONS: From the intersection of US 9 and NY 73/NY 74, near Exit 28 on I-87 N, head south on US 9. Turn left onto Alder Meadow Road at 0.6 miles. Follow Alder Meadow Road 2.1 miles, and bear left onto Crane Pond Road. The parking lot is on the left where the pavement ends, and Crane Pond Road turns into an unmaintained road at 1.4 miles.

GPS Parking Area Coordinates	17 Pharaoh Lake
UTM Zone (WGS 84):	18T
Easting:	0605376.4
Northing:	4857052.5
Latitude:	N 43° 51' 32.55"
Longitude:	W 73° 41' 19.54"

GPS Trailhead Coordinates	17 Pharaoh Lake
UTM Zone (WGS 84):	18T
Easting:	0607494.3
Northing:	4856227.2
Latitude:	N 43° 51' 4.70"
Longitude:	W 73° 39' 45.29"

18 Shelving Rock Falls

SCENERY: ✿ ✿ ✿ ✿	DISTANCE: *1.5 miles round-trip to falls,*
TRAIL CONDITION: ✿ ✿ ✿ ✿ ✿	*4.1 miles round-trip along lake*
CHILDREN: ✿ ✿ ✿ ✿ ✿	HIKING TIME: *2 hours*
DIFFICULTY: ✿	OUTSTANDING FEATURES: *Spectacular*
SOLITUDE: ✿ ✿	*waterfall, lakeside hiking, old foundation*

Following the shore of Lake George, the trail system around Shelving Rock Falls was once carriage roads and therefore makes for some of the easiest hiking in the Adirondacks. Though the trails are easy, they are beautiful and provide an excellent variety of scenery and history. You can explore the trails and destinations in a variety of ways, so consider the system of trails more of a destination than simply a hike.

Though many smaller parking areas are along Shelving Rock Road, the spaces are very limited, often with room for only one or two cars, and not clearly marked as parking areas. Because the entire roadside is plastered with signs warning that cars parked along the road will be towed, I would not plan on finding parking except in the large parking area for which the signs are obvious and directions are given. Likewise, trails leading to Lake George's shores are not clearly marked at the other parking areas, while the trail from the main parking area is impossible to miss.

On the right side of the parking area, walk past the vehicle barrier and down the broad access road. You have probably noticed that there is no trail register, nor are there any trail markers, but it is practically impossible to lose your way. Likewise, Shelving Rock Road and Lake George border the trail system, so you cannot wander far off the trail before regaining your bearings. Less than 0.3 miles in, you will come to a fork in the trail. Straight ahead is the main portion of the lakeside trails, while to your left are the falls. Continue to the left, and cross Shelving Rock Brook over a wooden bridge at

18 Shelving Rock Falls

N 0   0.1   0.2
        mile

Fourteenmile
Island

Shelving Rock
Mountain

Lake George

ADIRONDACK
STATE PARK

LAKE GEORGE
WILD FOREST

Shelving Rock Bay Trail

Shelving Rock Rd.

To
Hogtown
& 87

vehicle
barrier P

Log Bay
Island

waterfalls

Shelving Rock
Bay

old foundation

0.4 miles. On the opposite side of the bridge, you may notice a foot-path to your left. This footpath can be used to climb up to—or as your return route from—the falls. The stroll along the designated trail is an easier approach and has its own charms near the top.

You may have noticed that the trail system is more like a network of roads. Indeed, this area of Lake George Wild Forest was once a part of the Knapp Estate, and the trails were formerly carriage roads. The extensive work employed to level the terrain and build these roads becomes evident when you pass a large rock retaining wall on your left. The wall is part of a switchback that leads up the hill that eventually climbs to the top of Shelving Rock Falls. Tall pines thoroughly shade the area, and as you reach the height of the climb, you will notice a lone-wolf pine on your right.

Lone-wolf trees are trees that grow in open fields and eventually get overtopped when the forest takes over the field. Often short and gnarly, these trees eventually get shaded out and die, but they become excellent shelter and den trees. Any doubts that the environment has undergone a major transition are removed when you see the remains of a foundation behind the lone-wolf pine. This ruin adds an interesting spot for exploration, but the roar of the falls ahead will likely keep you from dallying long.

The carriage road takes you to the dam above the falls. Off to the right, the carriage road continues back to Shelving Rock Road, but straight ahead, you can make out the caissons that once supported a bridge over the artificial wetland that sprawls out before you. Across the dam, you can see a trail and might be tempted to cross the top of the dam, but do not attempt it. Bear in mind that the dam is narrow and covered in slick algae, and many people have been injured or have died here. The best and, coincidentally, most scenic way to reach the other side is at the base of the falls.

A short scramble downhill will take you there. Keep an eye out for a protruding rock on the right that makes an outstanding point to view and photograph the falls. The falls cascade 70 to 80 feet through and over large protrusions of ledge, with a deep pool beneath. You can return along the carriage road or take the more interesting foot-path down beside Shelving Rock Brook. Besides adding a little more interest to the hike, this path has the benefit of revealing another smaller falls about midway down to the bridge previously crossed. You will have to scramble along rocks and roots to get down, but the trail is no different from typical Adirondack trails.

Back on the trail, you have the option to head back to your vehicle, but it would be a shame to miss the excellent walk along Lake George that awaits you by continuing to your left at the first fork. The trail along the lakeshore is level, passes within feet of the lake for long portions, and has a few excellent lookouts. The trail ends at private property, and you can return to the parking lot along Shelving Rock Road, but the trail along the lake is so pleasant that it is by far your better option.

DIRECTIONS: From the intersection of NY 9/US 9 and NY 149, south of Lake George and north of Glen Lake, head east along NY 149. Turn left on Buttermilk Falls Road at 6 miles. Keep left at 3.1 miles, where Buttermilk Falls Road turns into Sly Pond Road. Sly Pond Road turns into Shelving Rock Road at 5.7 miles, just past the intersection with Hogtown Road on the right. Continue on Shelving Rock Road for 1.8 miles, where you pass the parking area for primitive campsites and register for the area. Continue to the left on Shelving Rock Road 1.8 miles to the parking area on your left.

GPS Trailhead Coordinates	18 Shelving Rock Falls
UTM Zone (WGS 84):	18T
Easting:	0612831.1
Northing:	4823503.0
Latitude:	N 43° 33' 21.42"
Longitude:	W 73° 36' 11.01"

19 Sleeping Beauty Mountain

SCENERY: ✿ ✿ ✿ ✿	DISTANCE: *3.3 or 4.4 miles*
TRAIL CONDITION: ✿ ✿ ✿ ✿	HIKING TIME: *2–3 hours*
CHILDREN: ✿ ✿ ✿ ✿ ✿	OUTSTANDING FEATURES: *Sheer cliffs,*
DIFFICULTY: ✿ ✿	*panoramic views*
SOLITUDE: ✿ ✿	

The sheer cliffs are a spectacle in and of themselves, but once you add the views of Lake George from Sleeping Beauty's summit, this becomes a must-visit trail. Though the hike is steep in sections, the short distance from Dacy Clearing places it easily within the grasp of hikers of all experience levels. A longer approach or additional circuit can be added for hikers who desire a more extensive adventure.

To reach the trailhead at Dacy Clearing, you can either drive or hike 1.6 miles from the Hogtown parking area. The road, though a bit narrow, is in good shape, and vehicles in good condition should have no difficulty reaching the clearing. This way passes multiple campsites, historic sites, and additional trailheads, so hikers wishing for additional interest or mileage may want to consider starting from the parking area.

Dacy Clearing has a large parking area, as well as some day-use facilities, including picnic tables and pit toilets, so don't be surprised to find many people who choose this as a destination in itself. The trailhead is in the southern corner of the parking area, just to the side of a vehicle barrier and stream. Yellow disks mark this portion of the trail. The trail heads southward but almost immediately switches back northward and begins a steady climb. The trail register is a few hundred yards from the switchback, and when you see how full the register is, it is obvious that this is a popular trail. The trail, wide enough for two to hike side by side, was once a part of the Knapp Estate's road network that weaves through the area. In 1931

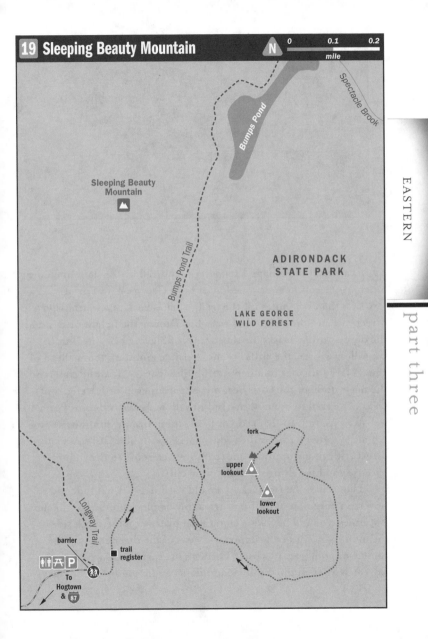

19 Sleeping Beauty Mountain

N

0   0.1   0.2
mile

EASTERN

part three

Bumps Pond

Spectacle Brook

Sleeping Beauty Mountain

Bumps Pond Trail

ADIRONDACK STATE PARK

LAKE GEORGE WILD FOREST

fork

upper lookout

lower lookout

Longway Trail

barrier

trail register

To Hogtown & 87

4,300 acres of the Knapp Estate were acquired by the state, including much of the southeastern section of Lake George Wild Forest.

Less than 0.5 miles in, the trail switches back in a southeastern direction, and the climb slackens a bit. During the height of summer, the dense canopy masks the sheer cliffs of Sleeping Beauty, but in the fall or winter, the cliffs are more visible and soon loom ahead of you. A large angular boulder at 0.6 miles marks a T in the trail, and the magnitude of the cliffs becomes apparent even with leafed-out trees. The trail to the left, marked in yellow, leads to Bumps Pond as well as a circuit trail that returns to Sleeping Beauty Summit, adding 1.8 miles to the trip. To the right, marked with blue disks, is a more direct and, in my opinion, more impressive route to the summit because you hike along the base of the cliffs.

The trail to the right leaves the old road network behind, and you traverse a narrow foot trail through a tiny hemlock grove. For the next 0.4 miles, you will be hiking along a flat plateau on the south side of the mountain, with truly impressive views of the sheer cliff and the tumble of boulders at its base. Through the surrounding canopy, you can catch brief glimpses of the mountains to the southwest, but they

View of lower lookout from upper lookout

don't compare to the vistas at the summit. The grade is basically flat, and though there are a few wet spots, it is easygoing. At 0.8 miles, you cross a 10-foot bridge, and the trail swings eastward. The trail dips down briefly, but at 1 mile, you begin the climb to the summit. Multiple switchbacks make the climb easier, and at 1.1 miles, you make your way up a substantially built-up switchback with a high rock wall.

After this point, the trail weaves its way northward on the east side of the cliffs, and views disappear as the forest becomes more coniferous. At 1.6 miles, you reach a Y in the trail. To the right is the trail to Bumps Pond and the circuit mentioned previously, while straight ahead is the summit, 0.1 mile. When you reach the end of the trail, you can view the panorama that opens out before you from several open ledges. Immediately in front of you is a large outcrop where people congregate; a higher but smaller outcrop is also to your right and slightly behind you, as well as a large lower one to the south. At the lower lookout, you have the advantage of seeing your path along the base of the cliffs. Expansive views to the west, south, and north show various portions of Lake George and the surrounding mountains from all of these lookouts, and there is plenty of room to sit and enjoy the views. Return the way you came for a total trip length of 3.6 miles, or take the circuit for a total length of 4.4 miles.

DIRECTIONS: From the intersection of NY 9/US 9 and NY 149 (south of Lake George and north of Glen Lake), head east along NY 149. Turn left on Buttermilk Falls Road at 6 miles. Keep left at 3.1 miles where Buttermilk Falls Road turns into Sly Pond Road. Sly Pond Road turns into Shelving Rock Road at 5.7 miles, just past the intersection with Hogtown Road on the right. Continue on Shelving Rock Road 1.8 miles to the Hogtown parking area. Park here if you desire a longer trip. Otherwise, continue down the one-lane road 1.6 miles to Dacy Clearing.

GPS Trailhead Coordinates	19 Sleeping Beauty Mountain
UTM Zone (WGS 84):	18T
Easting:	0616632.3
Northing:	4822853.9
Latitude:	N 43° 32' 58.28"
Longitude:	W 73° 33' 22.14"

20 Tongue Mountain Range

SCENERY: ✿ ✿ ✿ ✿
TRAIL CONDITION: ✿ ✿ ✿ ✿
CHILDREN: ✿
DIFFICULTY: ✿ ✿ ✿ ✿ ✿
SOLITUDE: ✿ ✿ ✿ ✿

DISTANCE: *12.6 miles (side trips not included)*
HIKING TIME: *8–10 hours*
OUTSTANDING FEATURES: *Multiple peaks with panoramic views, lakeside hiking, waterfall*

There are multiple ways to explore the Tongue Mountain Range, but this loop combines some of the best features into an extended day hike. Multiple peaks offer innumerable panoramic views of Lake George, as well as some pleasant hiking along old Civilian Conservation Corps (CCC) horse trails following the lakeshore. Along the ridgeline, there are few sources of water, so bring your own supply to drink.

🏃 Timber rattlesnakes are one of the few poisonous species of snakes found in New York and are seldom seen even in areas where they are known to live. The Tongue Mountain Range, as well as other areas along Lake George, is one of these few places and, though it is unlikely that you will encounter one, it is advisable to take precautions. See the section on animal hazards, page 17, and educate anyone unfamiliar with snakes. The simplest ways to avoid a mishap are to look where you step and to give the snake plenty of room should you see one.

The trailhead is a short distance south of the parking area along NY 9 N. Turn left onto the trail, marked in red, and you will find the trail register several hundred yards ahead. The trail descends through a stand of pines, and you pass what looks to be a fork in the trail on your left but is actually just a short footpath. Continue to your right downhill, and you soon reach a boardwalk that crosses the marsh surrounding Northwest Bay Brook. You reach a fork in the trail at 0.4 miles. To your right is the return leg of your trip along the Northwest Bay of Lake George, marked in blue. Continue straight,

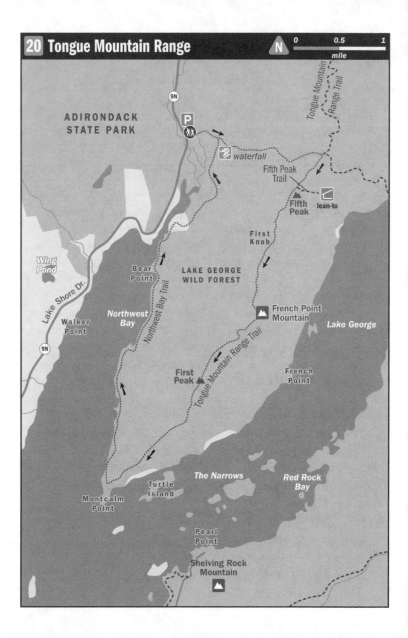

N

0   0.5   1

mile

ADIRONDACK
STATE PARK

9N

P

waterfall

Fifth Peak
Trail

Tongue Mountain Range Trail

Fifth
Peak

lean-to

First
Knob

Wing
Pond

Bear
Point

LAKE GEORGE
WILD FOREST

Lake Shore Dr.

Northwest Bay Trail

Northwest
Bay

Walker
Point

French Point
Mountain

Lake George

9N

Tongue Mountain Range Trail

First
Peak

French
Point

The Narrows

Red Rock
Bay

Turtle
Island

Montcalm
Point

Pearl
Point

Shelving Rock
Mountain

along the red-marked trail, which soon begins its ascent to the ridgeline. You will hear a waterfall off to your right shortly after the intersection. To view the 20-foot-high cascade, follow the barely discernible path on your right, or let the sounds of the falls guide you to the steep banks overlooking them.

The trail continues to climb, and you will cross and recross the seasonal stream that leads to the waterfall over log-and-plank bridges. The pitch has steadily increased, and soon steep ledges loom on your left. After walking in the shadow of these ledges, you make a final ascent over a built-up switchback to a brief plateau, a little less than 1 mile from the start. The approximate 0.3-mile stroll along the hemlock-shrouded plateau is a welcome break from the ascent, but you soon begin to climb again along a switchback. After more marshy areas and a little more climbing, you soon reach a four-way intersection, 2 miles. To your left, marked in blue, is the ridge trail north to Five Mile Mountain, Deer Leap, and the northern trailhead along NY 9 N. Straight ahead, marked in red, is the trail down to Five Mile Point on the shores of Lake George. Follow the blue-marked trail south, to your right, toward Fifth Peak, French Point

One of the many spectacular views along the Tongue Mountain Range

Mountain, and Montcalm Point along Lake George. The trip south is a bit like a roller coaster as you navigate up and down the numerous peaks and valleys that make up the dragon spine–like ridge.

The trail climbs the next 0.4 miles to where you reach the intersection with Fifth Peak Trail, marked in yellow. The summit is 0.3 miles along this spur. A lean-to is also located along this trail for those wishing to make it an overnight trip. There is no water, so campers should plan accordingly, as it is a steep climb to the lakeshore or any other source of water.

The trail continues straight, still marked in blue, around the west side of the mountain along a fairly level section. Views of the main portion of Lake George to the east are shortly followed with a view straight down to the Northwest Bay. The trail descends steeply after this point, and the roller coaster/sawteeth portion of the trail begins in earnest. After descending roughly 350 feet in less than 0.3 miles, you immediately begin to climb again to an unnamed knob, 3.6 miles to its top. This begins a series of steep ascents to fine views of the lake, followed by sharp descents. Each tiny summit provides an excellent place to stop, but if you plan on making only one stop along your traverse, I recommend waiting until you reach French Point Mountain, roughly 0.8 miles ahead after this first major descent. You scramble up, over, and down yet another knob, 4 miles, before you begin the final climb to French Point Mountain, 4.3 miles and 1,756 feet elevation. If you haven't taken in the beauty of the roughly 200 verdant green islands dotting the deep blue of Lake George, now is surely the time. The steep eastern side of the range has been swept with fire numerous times, and only scrubby trees dot the slope down to the lake, so panoramic views, open fields, and ledges are the norm and provide innumerable spots to stop.

You weave up and down another tiny knob and then see First Peak looming to the south. This peak is the last major dip and climb of the dragon's spine before the trail makes its last descent to Lake George at Montcalm Point. The trail descends approximately 500 feet before climbing another 300 feet over the next 1.4 miles on your way to First Peak, 5.7 miles from the start. Breathtaking views await you here, as well as along the majority of the descent to the lake. You are a little less than halfway through the hike, though you will have probably spent more than half of your planned time along the trail. Not to worry, the trail is mostly downhill or level as you complete the loop. Views of the Lake George Narrows sprawl out before you as you descend the mostly exposed portion of the tongue. Mileage to the innumerable vantage points would probably provide more confusion than any measure of progress. However, you reach the final knob approximately 0.5 miles after First Peak and, shortly after, delve back into the deeper woods. You reach the final intersection along the trail, 7.6 miles, at a wide and mucky area. To the left is Montcalm

Point, 0.2 miles, a welcome respite along the shores. Though the side trip is definitely worth a visit, those pressed for time can rest assured that numerous sections along the return trip traverse within feet of the lake and provide excellent points to stop and soak your feet or even take a swim.

To return, continue straight/right along the blue-marked trail northward. Shortly after the intersection, the trail passes within feet of the lake but soon arcs eastward into the forest to bypass a small section of private land. After this brief diversion, you rejoin the lakeshore and find that the trail generally follows the lake. The farther north you go, the better the condition of the trail and the easier the path. You pass several openings along the lake, along with stream crossings, abandoned fire pits, and swimming holes, so if time permits, enjoy the numerous points of interest, or plan to take a late-hike rest. Former CCC work is evident all along this return portion as you pass built-up crossings, rock walls, and other trail developments that make this portion of the trail truly a pleasure. At 10.6 miles, you reach the marsh where Northwest Bay Brook meets its namesake bay. It is only 1.6 miles back to the intersection and 2 miles to the parking area. An occasional passing truck along NY 9 N will remind you of this proximity, though the trail heads northeast into the forest a bit, and roadside noise is mostly drowned out. The trail climbs slightly during this 0.8-mile arc into the forest and soon descends back toward the marsh. Soon after the descent, you reach the trail intersection at 12.2 miles. Continue to the left back to your vehicle at the quarry-side parking area for a total trip of 12.6 miles (not including side trips).

View of Lake George

DIRECTIONS: From Exit 24 (CR 11/Bolton Landing/Riverbank Road) on I-87 N, head east on CR 11/Riverbank Road 4.7 miles. Turn left on NY 9 N/Lakeshore Drive, and head northeast 4.5 miles. The parking area is on your right in front of an old quarry.

GPS Trailhead Coordinates	**20 Tongue Mountain Range**
UTM Zone (WGS 84):	18T
Easting:	0612292.6
Northing:	4831368.4
Latitude:	N 43° 37' 43.59"
Longitude:	W 73° 36' 29.11"

N

0   5   10
miles

4

PART FOUR
Southern Hikes

21 Crane Mountain

SCENERY: 🌄 🌄 🌄 🌄	DISTANCE: *4.6 miles*
TRAIL CONDITION: 🌄 🌄 🌄	HIKING TIME: *5–6 hours*
CHILDREN: 🌄 🌄 🌄	OUTSTANDING FEATURES: *Panoramic view,*
DIFFICULTY: 🌄 🌄 🌄 🌄	*bald summit, pristine pond*
SOLITUDE: 🌄 🌄	

Crane Mountain is one of the most popular hikes in the southern Adirondacks: With its spectacular views and beautiful mountain pond, it is easy to see why. The climbing is steep, the descent bone–jarring, and the trail varied. It is a wonderful hike, but don't expect privacy, as dozens of groups visit the peak each day.

🚶 After the long, steep drive up the mountain along Ski Hi Road, you might begin to wonder how much climbing is left. The short answer is plenty; the trail climbs more than 1,100 feet in less than 0.8 miles. The climb is nearly vertical in sections, and you will have to use both hands in many places. Though it's certainly within the grasp of most hikers and many children, those with bad joints or balance won't find the climb or descent very enjoyable.

Head to the north end of the parking area, where you'll find the trail register a short distance up on your left. Stay to the right at the fork in the trail (to your left is the return leg), and begin climbing among mixed hardwoods. Approximately a quarter mile in, the vertical climb begins, and you have to pick your way over rough rocks and boulders. Because of the popularity of the trail, you will likely encounter other hikers along your way. There are many places to step off the trail to let others pass, and many of them are outlooks with outstanding views. At approximately 0.5 miles, the trail swings to the right, and you come out onto an open portion of ledge. Looking straight up the ledge, you will see a rock cairn that indicates where you pick up the trail again. At 0.7 miles, you come to a T; to your left is Crane Mountain

Pond, while the right leg is the Crane Mountain summit. The trail leads down, over a small hillock ahead, and then down again to the base of another vertical climb. At 0.8 miles, you come to the first of two wooden ladders that assist hikers over impassable vertical sections. After you climb the short ladder, the trail levels off briefly as it winds through stunted evergreens along the base of the summit's cliff. Chances are that you will see or, at the very least, hear other hikers who are sitting at the mountaintop. After heading east briefly, the trail switches back north, and you come to some steeper sections before the summit. A much longer ladder at 1.2 miles signals that the climb is nearly over. Upon reaching the summit at 1.4 miles, you will see numerous open sections along the cliff's edge. Hikers congregate here to enjoy the views and rest after the steep climb. There are plenty of places to rest, so if a section is occupied by another group, continue along the trail, and you will surely find a spot to yourself.

Along the peak, the trail weaves in and out of evergreens to the various lookouts along the cliff's edge. Many of these lookouts are visible from previous points, so you might want to leave someone behind to take a dramatic picture.

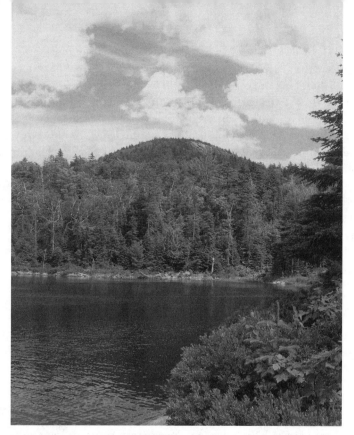

Looking back across Crane Mountain Pond

The climb down to Crane Mountain Pond is very steep and slippery and has the added hazard of many blown-down pines across the trail. Their whorls of broken branches make a veritable barricade of sharp stakes, so take your time making your way along this descent. The trail begins to level off when you reach a hardwood forest dominated by birches and maples. At 2.3 miles, you will come to a fork in the trail; straight ahead is a short path to an exposed boulder that sits above a wetland on Crane Mountain Pond's southeastern shore. From the fork, the main trail heads to your left and, after a brief foray into the woods, descends to the pond's shore. A fallen tree hides the trail along the shore, but undoubtedly you will have walked to the shore's edge to admire the view. Directly across a tiny bay in the pond is a sloping ledge that gradually enters the water. Hikers also congregate here, as it is popular for swimming. To reach this ledge, continue to your left along the shore through a small wet area and then though a dense coppice of cedars. Dragonflies will likely dive-bomb you through this section and as you step out onto the ledge. The spur back to the fork, at 0.7 miles, is near this sloped ledge. You can head back along it and then down the initial ascent to the parking area, if you choose not to follow the rest of the trail.

The trail continues to wind along the pond's shore and, after passing a small rocky bay on your right, crosses Putnam Brook. An arrow indicates that the trail continues to your left, but no mileage or details are given. The footpaths that head off in other directions are angler's paths or bushwhacks. Head west along the main trail, recross Putnam Brook, and come out onto a large, open portion of bedrock. There is no indication as to where the trail picks up again across this open rock face, but if you stick to the northern edge, next to Putnam Brook, you will find it. The trail begins to descend steeply again; be careful and take plenty of time along this stretch, as it is steeper—if you can believe it—than the ascent. The trail is very rocky, and you will likely need to crab-walk or scoot down several sections. Impressive views open up all over to the southwest, but keeping your eyes on the trail should be your main concern. The true path is often hard to discern because you traverse long sections of ledge or hop exclusively from boulder to boulder, both of which mask the footprints of previous hikers. Don't worry though; red DEC disks are clearly visible on the many maple trees that shade the trail. After 0.5 miles of descent, the trail levels off, and you will notice a small wetland to your left, around 3.2 miles. Shortly after, you cross over the stream that flows out of this wetland along a natural bridge. To either side of the bridge, you will see deep holes. Venturing to the rims of these holes reveals a water-carved cave underneath the bridge. Shortly after crossing, you descend to a feeder stream of Putnam Brook, as well as an intersection with the overgrown Crane Mountain Road. To your right, the road crosses the stream and enters private property, while to your left is a vehicle barrier and the return trip to the parking area. The abandoned road climbs steadily but gently through a mixed hardwood forest back to the parking area. The last mile of the hike is free of obstructions and easygoing, which is a welcome break from the more difficult ascent and descent. At 4.3 miles, you come to a fork where the road continues straight ahead and a trail heads off to the left. The trail leads to the register and north end of the parking lot. The road intersects Ski Hi Road a few hundred feet south of the parking area.

DIRECTIONS: In the hamlet of Thurman, head west on County Road 72/ Garnet Lake Road. Proceed 1.2 miles, and turn right onto Ski Hi Road. Ski Hi Road is a steep, rough dirt road, but it is maintained and drivable by most cars. Follow Ski Hi Road 1.8 miles, and bear right at the vehicle barrier. The road terminates at the parking area 0.1 mile past the barrier.

GPS Trailhead Coordinates	21 Crane Mountain
UTM Zone (WGS 84):	18T
Easting:	0583326.9
Northing:	4820975.1
Latitude:	N 43° 32' 13.46"
Longitude:	W 73° 58' 7.19"

22 Good Luck Cliffs

SCENERY: ✪ ✪ ✪ ✪ ✪	DISTANCE: *3.4 miles*
TRAIL CONDITION: ✪ ✪	HIKING TIME: *2–3 hours*
CHILDREN: ✪ ✪ ✪ ✪	OUTSTANDING FEATURES: *Dramatic cliffs,*
DIFFICULTY: ✪ ✪	*panoramic views*
SOLITUDE: ✪ ✪ ✪	

Sheer cliffs are almost standard in the High Peaks Region, but in the southern foot-hills, these dramatic cliffs are unique and rival those anywhere in the Adirondacks. Although the path to Good Luck Cliffs is technically a bushwhack, the cliffs are frequented enough that even in the height of winter, you can find your way to the mountaintop.

🚶🚶 The parking area is a few hundred yards north of the second bridge that crosses the West Branch of the Sacandaga River along NY 10 in the town of Arietta. Coming from the south, the parking area is a large pulloff on the right-hand side of the road.

The trailhead is across the street and has signs indicating that Dexter Lake is 4.1 miles, Potter Homestead is 7.1 miles, and Good Luck Lake is 0.4 miles, although the latter is along a separate trail. The trail register is approximately 0.5 miles ahead at a trail junction. Follow the snowmobile and red trail disks westward along mostly level terrain. Shortly after passing through a wet section, you reach the trail register and junction with other trails. To the right is a snowmobile trail that parallels NY 10. Straight ahead is the trail to Dry and Dexter lakes, 1.6 and 2.4 miles respectively. The left trail takes you to the west shore of Good Luck Lake (including some tent sites), Spectacle Lake, and the unmarked path to the cliffs and Good Luck Mountain summit.

The trail has several muddy and wet sections as you make your way southward toward the lake, and it even shares space with a stream for a while. The trail begins to descend from this junction,

N

0   0.15   0.3
mile

SOUTHERN

part four

To
Arietta

Chub Lake

W. Branch Sacandaga River

W. Branch Sacandaga River

P

To
Piseco

W. Branch Sacandaga River

Good Luck Lake

W. Stoner Lake Trail

trail
register

FERN'S LAKE
WILD FOREST

ADIRONDACK
STATE PARK

State Brook

Dexter Lake Trail

W. Stoner Lake Trail

boulder
cave

and at approximately 1 mile in, the lake comes into view. A designated campsite to the left of the trail provides an excellent point to view the lake. The cliffs soon become visible, looming off to your right, and you continue past the western tip of the lake through a marshy area, where the evergreens become denser. After crossing a short bridge, you reach the crest of a tiny hill, at 1.3 miles, below which is another bridge that crosses a stream that feeds Good Luck Lake. To your right is the unmarked path that leads to the cliffs.

The path parallels the feeder stream briefly on your left, along an elevated knoll, before swinging northwest toward the cliffs. Shortly after, the trail climbs and you rock-hop across a stream that cuts the gorge along the cliff's southwest face. The path follows within a few hundred feet of this stream all the way to a notch that lies just below the cliffs. In winter, icicles form sheets of ice along the southern tumble of boulders, creating an amazing winter wonderland setting.

Though the cliffs have been visible through most of the climb, their full grandeur is not fully expressed until you reach the small saddle beneath the west face of the cliff. The trail swings northward here, and you will navigate your way around a jumble of boulders

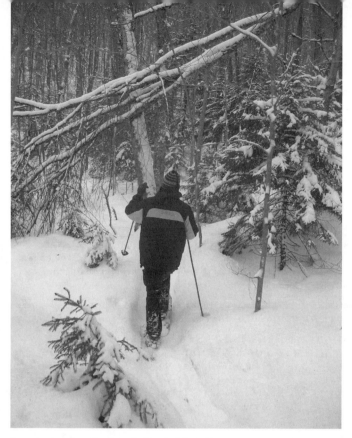

Snowshoeing along the unmarked part of the trail

that covers the valley floor. The huge boulders provide an excellent opportunity for exploration, including many small caves that are formed in the mass of rock. You pass a noteworthy cave on the right of the trail at 1.4 miles.

You probably have heard the stream flowing on your right, and at 1.5 miles, you recross it before the final ascent to the cliff top. The trail is much steeper and the path less distinct, but as long as you keep the cliffs to your right, you will eventually make your way to the north, or back, side of the cliffs. About 0.1 mile from the stream crossing, you reach a fork in the trail in a stand of spruce trees. To the left is a slight northward jog in the trail that leads to the summit, while the right trail leads to the summit a little more steeply but more directly. Either way, you reach the summit shortly; from there, take any of the numerous paths that weave their way from outlook to outlook. Along the southwest edge is a particularly amazing vista that shows expansive views down to the valley, with Spectacle Lake in the foreground.

DIRECTIONS: *From the south* From the intersection of NY 29–A and NY 10, north of Caroga Lake, head north on NY 10 6 miles. The large parking area is on the right just past the second bridge crossing the Sacandaga River in the town of Arietta.

From the north From the intersection of NY 8 and NY 10 in Piseco, head south on NY 10 11.6 miles. The large parking area is on your left.

GPS Trailhead Coordinates	22 Good Luck Cliffs
UTM Zone (WGS 84):	18T
Easting:	0537393.9
Northing:	4789199.0
Latitude:	N 43° 15' 21.19"
Longitude:	W 74° 32' 21.56"

23 Groff Creek

SCENERY: ⭐ ⭐ ⭐	DISTANCE: *5 miles*
TRAIL CONDITION: ⭐ ⭐ ⭐	HIKING TIME: *3–4 hours*
CHILDREN: ⭐ ⭐ ⭐	OUTSTANDING FEATURES: *Two unique*
DIFFICULTY: ⭐ ⭐	*waterfalls*
SOLITUDE: ⭐ ⭐ ⭐ ⭐ ⭐	

The two unique waterfalls along Groff Creek make this a must–experience trip for waterfall lovers. Though technically a bushwhack (the trail is unmarked), it is very easy to follow all the way to the marsh at the end.

🥾 The trail is at the end of the maintained section of River Road. The trail continues along this road briefly, but a sign warns that the road farther on is abandoned and you are proceeding at your own risk. Park along the pullout to the west of this sign, and make your way north along the broad, flat road. The road parallels the Sacandaga River and provides pleasant views of it. At 0.2 miles, you will pass a designated camping area on your right that is encircled by tall pines and provides ample room to set up. Views of the river are limited from this site. Shortly past the designated campsite, you will see the remains of an old stone foundation on your left. A little more than 0.3 miles along the road, you pass the posts for an old vehicle barrier and then a small white building on your left. A wooden bridge crosses Pete's Creek just past this building. Approximately 0.3 miles after the bridge, you reach an intersection in the road. Continue straight on the right-hand side of the fork another 0.1 mile, where you reach Forest Preserve lands.

You will pass a pulloff along the road on your left and then a small parking area at 0.8 miles. This marks the end of the road and the farthest point reached by vehicle if you should chance the abandoned road. The trail to your left still follows an old

N

0   0.2   0.4
mile

Scribner Hill Rd.

30

River Rd.

To
Northville
& Gloversville

P

Sacandaga River

30

stone
foundation

white
building

fork

pulloff

River Rd.

Pete's Creek

Groff Creek

◀ Groff
Mountain

waterfall

waterfall

SILVER LAKE
WILDERNESS

ADIRONDACK
STATE PARK

logging road, but nature has reclaimed much of it, and only a narrow footpath remains. The trail begins to climb for the next 0.5 miles as you work your way to the north side of Groff Mountain. The terrain falls off steeply on your right down to Groff Creek, and about 1.8 miles from the start, you will glimpse the first waterfall along the creek. There is no clear path down to view the waterfall, so pick your way carefully down the hillside and through the tall hemlocks to the top of the falls. The banks of the creek surrounding the waterfall are extremely steep on this side, but if you make your way to the top of the falls, you can cross to the other side and then zigzag your way down to the base. The nearly 30-foot vertical drop ends in a shallow pool, which is surrounded on three sides with vertical walls. Inside this natural amphitheater, the tumble of the falls drowns out all other sounds.

The second waterfall along this section of the creek is 0.1 mile farther west along the trail. Unlike the previous waterfall, this one is visible from the trail. Similar to the first one, no distinguishable path leads to it, though the route down is less steep. A frothy cascade, this waterfall steps its way down a series of ledges to a shallow

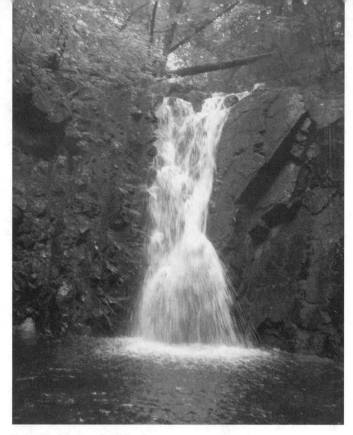

First waterfall along Groff Creek

pool as well. Downstream are a series of flumes and cascades that add waterscapes of their own.

While exploring these falls, you are in prime habitat of the red-spotted newt. The adult newt is olive green with red spots along its back, but you are far more likely to encounter and recognize it in its terrestrial juvenile stage. The juvenile, known as a red eft, is brilliant orange with red dots and is common in woodlands near creeks and streams.

The trail continues another 0.5 miles west to where the creek levels off and a marsh is formed. It continues along the south side of the marsh, though where it truly ends is hard to discern. Another set of waterfalls is said to be found on the opposite shore if you follow a tributary stream around a major bend. This would require serious bushwhacking, as there is no clear path. I attempted to find them during a heavy rain but soon decided to leave their discovery for another expedition. Return back along the path for a total trip length of 5 miles.

DIRECTIONS: *From the south*   From the intersection of NY 30 and NY 30-A in Gloversville, head north on NY 30 13.6 miles, and turn left on County Road 6. Just after crossing the Sacandaga River, turn right onto River Road. Follow River Road north 4.6 miles to where the signs warn that the road is abandoned. Park to the left of the road.

From the north   From the intersection of NY 30 and NY 8 in Wells, head south on NY 30 15.8 miles, and turn left on CR 6. Just after crossing the Sacandaga River, turn right onto River Road. Follow River Road north 4.6 miles to where the signs warn that the road is abandoned. Park to the left of the road.

GPS Trailhead Coordinates	23 Groff Creek
UTM Zone (WGS 84):	18T
Easting:	0560275.8
Northing:	4795922.3
Latitude:	N 43° 18' 49.40"
Longitude:	W 74° 15' 24.13"

24 Hadley Mountain

SCENERY: ☘ ☘ ☘ ☘	DISTANCE: *3.6 miles*
TRAIL CONDITION: ☘ ☘ ☘	HIKING TIME: *2–3 hours*
CHILDREN: ☘ ☘ ☘ ☘	OUTSTANDING FEATURES: *Panoramic views,*
DIFFICULTY: ☘ ☘	*fire tower*
SOLITUDE: ☘	

A short and steady climb to the top of this 2,680-foot bald summit provides great views of the southern Adirondacks. With a climbable fire tower, summertime summit steward, and a broad, open mountaintop ideal for a picnic, Hadley Mountain is an excellent choice for family outings.

🚶🚶 The trailhead parking area accommodates dozens of hikers, but the popularity of the trail means that you will likely have to park on the side of the dirt access road. The trailhead is clearly marked with a painted DEC sign, as well as a historical marker describing the history of the fire tower. Several fires at the opening of the 20th century swept the area, and most of the forest, including the topsoil, was burned off. A wooden tower was erected in 1916, according to a placard, but other sources date it to 1917. After blowing over in severe winds, a steel tower was re-erected with guylines in 1920. Because the risk of forest fires in the Adirondacks is generally negligible, the use of fire towers for fire suppression has given way to aerial observation; consequently the tower, cabin, and trail fell into disrepair. However, within the past couple of decades, the Hadley Mountain Fire Tower Committee has restored the tower, cabin, and trail, and the old observer's cabin is now manned daily from the Fourth of July until Labor Day by a tower steward. According to the DEC Unit Management Plan, the steward is also available on weekends through Columbus Day.

The beginning of the trail is surrounded by a thick stand of hemlocks that continues to provide shade up to the trail register, where

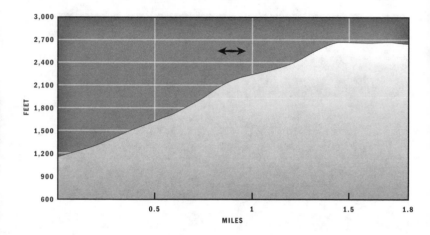

the evergreens give way to a mainly beech and birch forest that is thick with saplings and shades the trail for most of the climb. The trail, marked by red DEC trail markers, begins to ascend immediately and continues steadily uphill for nearly I mile, where it levels off for a while before the final climb to the summit. Over this first section, large rocks and cobbles are strewn across many portions, while other parts proceed up bare bedrock. Chances are that you will need to step off the trail frequently, as many hikers will be either ascending or descending. The trail is so clear that directions are hardly needed.

Upon reaching the ridgeline, views to the southeast glimpsed through the canopy hint at the truly panoramic views that await you shortly ahead. Along the ridgeline, the flora is mostly scrubby trees or saplings, and the trail is mostly clear of the rocks and cobbles that covered the path previously. You will pass through a small notch in the bedrock, followed by a sharp turn left before the last climb to the summit. The mountaintop is almost entirely exposed bedrock with many places to sit and enjoy the views. In fact, when I reached the summit, there were more than a dozen families or groups, with ample room for people to spread out to enjoy an afternoon picnic. Panoramic views in all directions are available, and you can see even farther into the surrounding country if you climb the fire tower. To the southwest, you can see Great Sacandaga Lake; to the north, some of the famous High Peaks; to the south, glimpses of the Catskills; and to the east, the foothills surrounding Lake George and even the Green Mountains of Vermont or the Berkshires in Massachusetts. A steady breeze helps to keep the infamous black flies at bay, and with the spectacular views, it is clear why this is a popular picnic spot for families.

DIRECTIONS: Heading north on NY 9 N, cross the Sacandaga River and turn left on School Street. Continue straight onto Bridge Street. Cross the Hudson River, and keep left onto County Road 4/Rockwell Street. Turn right onto CR 1/Stony Creek Road, approximately 0.5 miles from your turn onto School Street. Head north on CR 1, and keep left at 3.1 miles onto Hadley Hill Road. Continue along Hadley Hill Road for 2.7 miles, and turn right on Eddy Road. Keep left on Tower Road (dirt road) at 0.8 miles. Tower Road heads north, swings west, and then curves back south. At 1.7 miles, the trailhead parking area is on the right.

GPS Trailhead Coordinates	24 Hadley Mountain
UTM Zone (WGS 84):	18T
Easting:	0585018.6
Northing:	4802848.0
Latitude:	N 43° 22' 25.27"
Longitude:	W 73° 57' 2.00"

25 Jockeybush Lake

SCENERY: ✿ ✿ ✿	DISTANCE: *2.3 miles*
TRAIL CONDITION: ✿ ✿ ✿	HIKING TIME: *2 hours*
CHILDREN: ✿ ✿ ✿ ✿ ✿	OUTSTANDING FEATURES: *Pristine lake,*
DIFFICULTY: ✿ ✿	*waterfall*
SOLITUDE: ✿ ✿ ✿ ✿	

Another one of the short hikes featured in the book, Jockeybush Lake promises a varied experience, from streamside hiking and crossings to lakeside camping and even a small waterfall. As with other short hikes, this one promises a great experience for beginning hikers and a pleasant trip for the whole family. During the spring thaw, Jockeybush Outlet may require wading, so plan accordingly.

🚶 Parking for Jockeybush Lake is a pulloff on the west side of NY 10, just across from Lake Alma. Essentially a pond, Lake Alma has a large painted black-and-white sign with a green pine tree that is clearly visible when approaching from the south. Coming from the north, keep an eye out for the DEC trail signs.

The trail begins in the northwest corner of the pulloff, and the trail register is a few yards along the path. The trail is well marked with blue trail disks and has no intersections, so finding your way is straight-forward. Roughly 0.3 miles in, you cross a seasonal stream that has a few mucky spots, and you will likely have to find a crossing off the trail. You will soon see Jockeybush Outlet flowing on your left and will cross to its southern bank across a rocky wash. During summer this crossing will barely break your stride, but during times of high water, you may have to wade. Shortly after crossing the outlet, you pass a small waterfall on your right that feeds into the outlet. The cascade weaves its way down moss-covered ledges into a verdant jumble of rocks. You can rock-hop around and eventually scramble to the top of the cascade some dozen feet above the outlet to see another tiny cascade.

25 Jockeybush Lake

N

| 0 | 0.25 | 0.5 |

mile

To Piseco

Teeter Creek

10

Pine Mountain

To Arietta

10

Jockeybush Outlet

Lake Alma

P trail register

small stream crossing

waterfall

Kennels Pond

FERN'S LAKE WILD FOREST

ADIRONDACK STATE PARK

Jockeybush Outlet

Ely Mountain

Limestone Creek

Iron Lake

Jockeybush Lake

SOUTHERN

part four

After the short diversion at the falls, the trail weaves its way along the southern banks of the outlet for the rest of the way to Jockeybush Lake, almost without incident. The one exception is a long muddy section, about a mile in, that fills the entire trail. You'll have to either traverse the muck or bypass along one of the newer footpaths that hikers have made. As is the case with most trails, it is best to minimize your impact on the surrounding forest by following a path already worn by previous hikers than tramping along undisturbed areas. Soon after the mire, you will find yourself on the eastern end of Jockeybush Lake. The lake is deep, as far as Adirondack lakes are concerned, but it's not readily apparent at this end, as it is shallow here. Bushwhacks along either shore reveal that the lake is deeper than it first appears. At this end of the lake, a logjam forms a dam, as well as a means to the opposite bank of the outlet, where a designated campsite is situated in a small stand of hemlocks. The campsite has admirable views westward along the fingerlike lake and is an ideal spot to camp or picnic during a day trip. Numerous footpaths diverge from the end of the trailhead and campsite, promising other vantage points and even a prime

Jockeybush Lake as seen from the campsite on its eastern tip

swimming spot, but the trail described ends here. Return the way you came for a round-trip of 2.3 miles.

DIRECTIONS: *From the south*   From the intersection of NY 29-A and NY 10, north of Caroga Lake, head north on NY 10, and continue 9.6 miles. The parking area is on the left, opposite Lake Alma, and has a large black-and-white sign.

From the north   From the intersection of NY 8 and NY 10 in Piseco, head south on NY 10, and continue 7.9 miles. The large parking area is on your right, opposite Lake Alma.

GPS Trailhead Coordinates	25 Jockeybush Lake
UTM Zone (WGS 84):	18T
Easting:	0535215.0
Northing:	4794327.4
Latitude:	N 43° 18' 3.43"
Longitude:	W 74° 33' 57.00"

26 Stewart and Indian Lakes

SCENERY: ✿ ✿ ✿	SOLITUDE: ✿ ✿ ✿ ✿ ✿
TRAIL CONDITION: ✿ ✿ ✿ ✿	DISTANCE: *4.6 miles*
CHILDREN: ✿ ✿ ✿ ✿ ✿	HIKING TIME: *2–3 hours*
DIFFICULTY: ✿	OUTSTANDING FEATURES: *Two secluded lakes*

This easy hike is a great destination for people who wish to explore two remote, picturesque lakes for fishing or a picnic. With a few moderate climbs, it is a good trail for children, and excellent wildlife viewing at both lakes provides additional interest.

🚶🚶 Located in the Shaker Mountain Wild Forest, the trail utilizes old logging roads, so the grades are mostly gentle and easily accessible to hikers of all experience levels. The area had been heavily logged before state acquisitions, and much of the forest is still in a phase of regeneration. However, the acquisitions occurred decades ago, and traces of past logging have disappeared. Wild forest areas—in contrast to wilderness, primitive, or canoe areas—are considered less ecologically fragile, allowing for a greater variety of uses and more intensive activities. Don't let the distinction fool you, though, as they are definitely wild places and provide excellent wilderness experiences. Access to the parking area is at the left fork along Green Lake Road, which appears to be little more than a driveway. The well-maintained and spacious lot provides parking for the Kane Mountain Trail as well, but the lot can easily accommodate a dozen cars, so space should not be a concern.

The trail begins to the right of the trail register on the north end of the parking lot. Shrouded in tall pines, the trail follows an access road to a small fish hatchery. The damming of Otter Lake's outlet created the hatchery, and you can hear water spilling over the concrete dam in most seasons. The trail diverges from the road shortly before the pond on your right. The exact path may be a little hard to discern, but a sign prohibiting the use of baitfish and a wooden bridge will steer you.

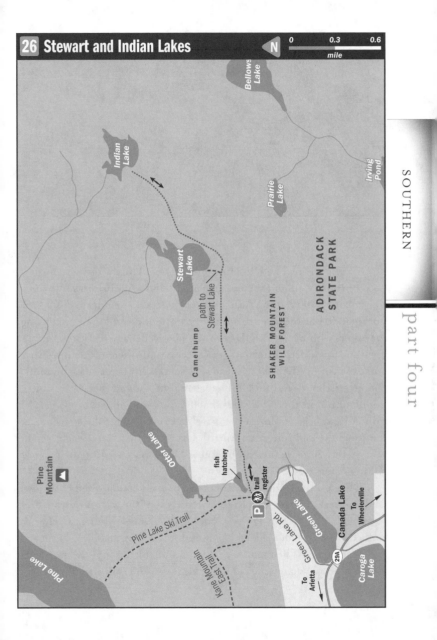

N

| 0 | 0.3 | 0.6 |

mile

Bellows Lake

Indian Lake

Irving Pond

Prairie Lake

Stewart Lake

path to Stewart Lake

Camelhump

SHAKER MOUNTAIN WILD FOREST

ADIRONDACK STATE PARK

Otter Lake

Pine Mountain

fish hatchery

trail register

Pine Lake

Pine Lake Ski Trail

P

Kane Mountain East Trail

Green Lake Rd.

Green Lake

To Arietta

Canada Lake

To Wheelerville

29A

Caroga Lake

SOUTHERN

part four

A note to anglers: The DEC has gone to great lengths to reestablish native brook trout and the endangered round whitefish in some of the isolated waters of the Adirondacks. Reestablishment methods vary but include poisoning entire lakes with rotenone and then restocking the waters with native fish. Due to the physical characteristics of the various Adirondack waterways, the success of this technique is limited and expensive. When the technique is successful, those same physical characteristics mean there will be lasting success and that native fish populations can thrive. Unfortunately, the reintroduction of nonnative species is almost exclusively a consequence of the unintentional use and release of baitfish by anglers into the reestablished ecosystems. So leave the bait bucket at home when visiting the prized fishing waters of the Adirondacks.

Once on the trail, you will notice that it is emblazoned by yellow trail markers and very easy to follow the rest of the way. A quick climb takes you along a low ridge overlooking the pond to your left. The trail climbs through a mixed hardwood forest dominated by birch and beech trees. The grade is very moderate for the first 0.7 miles, at which point you encounter a muddy area. The trail climbs more steeply after this muddy area, but at approximately 1.2 miles, it levels off to a more gently rolling terrain. Farther along the trail, the forest canopy gets higher and the understory thins, allowing deeper views into the surrounding forest. You catch glimpses of Stewart Lake as you approach 1.3 miles, where there is a fork in the trail. The main trail continues on the right toward Indian Lake, while the left fork takes you through a stand of pine and hemlock to a boggy area that surrounds Stewart Lake. The marshland prevents you from gaining direct access to the lake but makes for good wildlife viewing.

Back along the trail, you encounter some mucky areas that you will have to negotiate on your own, as no good way bypasses the muck. At 2 miles, you pass a thick carpet of club moss, which at first glance looks like tree saplings but is actually more closely related to ferns. At this point, you begin the descent to Indian Lake, where the trail ends at the shore. A path to the left follows the shoreline toward a rock that juts out into the lake and provides additional vantage points. The remote setting promises an excellent opportunity to view a variety of wildlife, including a beaver lodge.

DIRECTIONS: From the southern intersection of NY 10 and NY 29-A in Caroga Lake, head north on NY 10/NY 29-A. At 3.4 miles past the intersection, turn right onto Green Lake Road. From the north and west, head south on NY 10/NY 29-A, and turn left at 1.9 miles past the northern intersection of NY 10 and NY 29-A. Follow Green Lake Road north along the west edge of the shore. At 0.5 miles, bear left onto the parking area drive.

GPS Trailhead Coordinates	26 Stewart and Indian Lakes
UTM Zone (WGS 84):	18T
Easting:	0540235.1
Northing:	4780903.5
Latitude:	N 43° 10' 47.37"
Longitude:	W 74° 30' 17.72"

27 Tenant Creek Falls

SCENERY: ✿ ✿ ✿ ✿	DISTANCE: *4.2 miles*
TRAIL CONDITION: ✿ ✿ ✿	HIKING TIME: *3–4 hours*
CHILDREN: ✿ ✿ ✿ ✿	OUTSTANDING FEATURES: *Three unique*
DIFFICULTY: ✿ ✿	*waterfalls*
SOLITUDE: ✿ ✿ ✿ ✿	

Reaching the first of these three beautiful and distinct waterfalls is easy. Its cascading waters over exposed rock faces are impressive and sure to please. Finding the second and third falls requires a bit of bushwhacking along a maze of paths, but the two serene and Zen-like waterfalls are excellent compensation.

👫 Access to the three falls is along a trail that initially passes through private property. Please respect the property by staying on the marked trail for the first 0.5 miles and by not blocking the road or parking in front of the vehicle-barrier gate. As with many trails in the Adirondacks, access to some of the park's most interesting features is available through the cooperation of private landholders; by keeping up our end of the bargain, we can ensure that access to these gems is available in the future.

The trail begins to the left of the parking area and heads north along East Stony Creek. The trail register is just inside the trailhead, and you will have to negotiate a few muddy spots along this brief portion of the trail. At 0.2 miles, Tenant Creek, spanned by a large wooden bridge, empties into East Stony Creek. The trail across the bridge leads to Wilcox Lake via the aptly named East Stony Creek Trail. A painted sign indicates that the falls are to your right and to the east up Tenant Creek. You will pass numerous signs and arrows indicating that the trail is next to the creek, and reminding that you are still on private property.

You will be following Tenant Creek to each of the falls, but this portion of the trail is an old logging road and is the easiest section to

N

0   0.2   0.4
mile

SOUTHERN

part four

ADIRONDACK
STATE PARK

WILCOX LAKE
WILD FOREST

waterfalls

Tenant Creek

waterfall

Tenant Creek Falls Trail

Rand
Mountain

To
Bakertown

E. Stony Creek Trail

Mudcreek Rd.

wooden
bridge

E. Stony Creek

trail register

vehicle
barrier

P

Mudcreek Rd.

To
Northville

follow. With a clear path underfoot, you will find plenty of opportunities to look out on the boulder-strewn creek. After crossing a
distinct wet area, you will climb away from the creek onto a ridge. By
now, the roar of the falls is distinct and loud just ahead, and you will
likely leave the trail to scrabble among the myriad paths that weave
down to the base of the falls.

Tumbling over a sloping rock face, water falls 50 feet into a large
basin at the foot of the falls. Tall hemlocks frame the pool, and numerous boulders along its rocky shore provide excellent places to stop and
contemplate the scene. This is likely as far as many visitors come because
the trail—or more accurately, path—is less distinct and practically disappears on occasion as it winds upstream. However, it's hardly a problem,
as your destination is along this creek. If you follow it upstream and keep
it on your left, you will find the second and third falls.

Scramble back up to the top of the falls, and begin to pick your
way along the creek bank. The transition from trail to multiple paths is
at its worst at this point, so stay close to the creek and you will eventually find the trail again. Though it is not difficult, you will have to be
nimble to pick your way through the rocks and tangle of roots. The

creek forms a small bulge, or horseshoe, around 1.2 miles, after which the flow levels off and the banks become grassy. Shortly after, you will cross a tiny stream around 1.3 miles, and then the trail climbs slightly uphill away from the creek. The trail follows an elevated ridge briefly and then descends to the creek again. After crossing and recrossing a tiny branch of the creek, you come out on a ledge across from the second falls, which cascade into a broad pool before you. I noticed many salamanders in the pool around the remains of crayfish.

The third falls is a few hundred yards upstream, with the best view from a sloped boulder next to the trail. Both falls are small, but the sheer rock ledges and encroaching forest make each feel wild and isolated. The pools at the bases are deep and enclosed, making excellent spots to take a swim. The roaring of the falls in their mini amphitheaters resonates deeply and drowns out the sounds of the surrounding forest. It is very easy to be drawn in and enchanted by these serene and wild places, so plan to spend some extra time to enjoy the solitude.

DIRECTIONS: From the intersection of County Road 6 and NY 30 in Northville, head north along NY 30. After crossing the Sacandaga River, turn right onto CR 15/Old Northville Road. Continue on Old Northville Road 1.4 miles, and turn left onto East Stony Creek Road. (Some maps show this road as Mudcreek Road, Mason Road, CR 7, or Hope Falls Road, but local signs designate it as East Stony Creek Road.) Follow East Stony Creek Road (dirt road) past several designated primitive campsites to the parking area at 7.4 miles. Do not block the vehicle-barrier gate.

GPS Trailhead Coordinates	27 Tenant Creek Falls
UTM Zone (WGS 84):	18T
Easting:	0565985.8
Northing:	4799875.5
Latitude:	N 43° 20' 55.81"
Longitude:	W 74° 11' 8.96"

Northern Hikes (28–33)

N

0   5   10
miles

Moose Mountain
Lake Placid
Lake Placid
3
Vermontville

Essex County
Franklin County

86
Saranac Lake

Santanoni Peak

Newcomb

3
Lower Saranac Lake

28N

Paul Smiths
Lake Clear
Lake Clear
33
30
Upper Saranac Lake
29

Long Lake

Saint Regis River

30
Tupper Lake

Long Lake
32
30

Mount Matumbla
Tupper Lake

Franklin County
Hamilton County

W. Branch Saint Regis River

3

Raquette River
Childwold

ADIRONDACK STATE PARK

Carry Falls Reservoir
56

Cranberry Lake
Cranberry Lake

S. Branch Grass River

3

Hamilton County
Herkimer County

Saint Lawrence County

28-30

Wanakena

31   CR 27

Alder Bed Mountain

5

PART FIVE
Northern Hikes

SCENERY: ☆ ☆ ☆ ☆	DISTANCE: *9.7 miles, 4.8 miles by boat*
TRAIL CONDITION: ☆ ☆ ☆ ☆	HIKING TIME: *5–6 hours*
CHILDREN: ☆ ☆	OUTSTANDING FEATURES: *Scenic pond,*
DIFFICULTY: ☆ ☆ ☆	*beautiful vistas*
SOLITUDE: ☆ ☆ ☆ ☆	

Cat Mountain is a beautiful little peak that offers excellent views. Combined with the High Falls overnight trip, it makes a nice side trip or an extended day trip on its own. To add a bit more adventure to the hike, you can boat in from Cranberry Lake to Janacks Landing and bypass roughly 5 miles of the round-trip hike.

🚶 Hike in from the western terminus of the High Falls Loop in Wanakena or by boating into Janacks Landing in the Dead Creek Flow arm of Cranberry Lake. The trail described here will be from Wanakena with a side note about boating access, but boaters can pick up the trail and follow the description from the Janacks Landing intersection.

The trail and register are elevated a few feet above the spacious parking area on the southern edge. The trail begins heading easterly but quickly swings south along an abandoned logging road. The wide and flat roadbed, over relatively level terrain, allows for easy hiking for the first 2 miles. You will make quick time, except where flooding due to beaver activity inundates the trail. You will encounter several mires, as well as sections of knee-deep water. The nearly black, murky waters are deceptive; although most of the time the water is less than 1 inch deep when it flows over the berms and beaver dams, occasional breaks in dams and the soft mud underfoot lead to drops of 1 foot or more, with little evidence provided by the placid waters. Hiking sticks act as excellent probes in doubtful waters and, as is the case at most trail-heads, previous hikers typically leave decent ones at the trail register.

N

0   0.5   1
mile

NORTHERN

part five

Olmstead Pond

Simmons Pond

Smile Creek Trail

Smile Creek

Cowhorn Pond

Big Deer Pond Trail

weather station

Cat Mountain

Cat Mountain Pond

Cowhorn Junction Trail

Dead Creek Flow

Janacks Landing

Glasby Pond

Sand Hill Trail

FIVE PONDS WILDERNESS

Dead Creek

Roundtop Mountain

South Shore Rd.

Ranger School Rd.

CR 61

To 3 & Cranberry Lake

Skate Creek

P

ADIRONDACK STATE PARK

The road, emblazoned with red disks, gently descends most of the way, and at approximately 1.5 miles, the waters of Dead Creek Flow become visible. The road closely follows the shoreline for 0.4 miles, at which point you come across a large campsite. Boaters often use this and the other 46 designated primitive sites along the lakeshore. At this point, the road ends, and the trail becomes a typical Adirondack trail. It crosses Dead Creek at 2.3 miles and then swings around the bay of Dead Creek Flow and heads east for 0.5 miles.

After the short easterly jog along the trail, you reach the intersection of the Janacks Landing Trail. The trail is now heading nearly due south and gradually climbs to Sand Hill Junction. The climb is steady and crisscrosses a small stream in several places before reaching the junction at 3.6 miles. Straight ahead is the easterly leg of the High Falls Loop, while the Cat Mountain summit and Glasby Pond are to your left along the Cowhorn Junction Trail.

The trail, marked with yellow disks, climbs steadily along Glasby Creek past a few small cascades, and the rush of water on your right is a pleasant addition to the trail. After passing through a small bramble-filled meadow, you come out on the western shores of

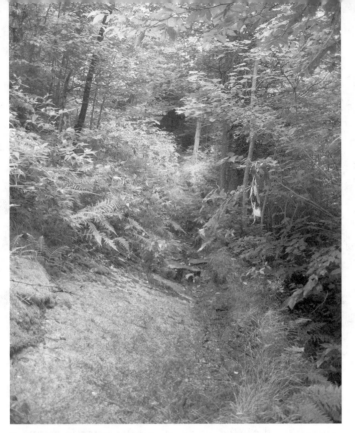

Section of trail before Glasby Pond

Glasby Pond at 3.8 miles. The steep cliffs of Cat Mountain provide a striking view across the pristine waters. You will pass through a large campsite before weaving your way up and over a tiny hillock, after which the pondside trail becomes a continuous mire. The terrain grows steadily steeper as you head away from the pond, and you soon reach the final fork in the trail. The Cowhorn Junction Trail continues off to your right toward Cowhorn and Cat Mountain ponds,

Glasby Pond

marked by yellow disks; to reach the Cat Mountain summit, veer to your left and follow the red trail markers.

The next 0.6 miles to the summit are the steepest sections, and the trail is a mix of short scrambles over bedrock and boulder-strewn steps. The hardwoods at the base of the mountain give way to wind-swept evergreens as you weave your way through small switchbacks. Paths on the left reach a few rocky outlooks. These offer nice views, but the best are available at the summit. The trail finally winds its way out onto the southern cliff tops. You'll find a solar-powered weather station and the remnants of an old fire tower here at the trail end. Enjoy excellent views on this portion of the cliffs, or search for better ones by dipping into the coppice of evergreens behind you and making your way along paths to the next section of the cliff top. The drop-off to the south is quite sheer, which allows spectacular views down to Cat Mountain Pond as well as Roundtop and Threemile mountains along the horizon.

Side note about boat access: A public boat launch is located just off of NY 3, on Columbian Road near Cranberry Lake's dam in the village of Cranberry Lake. The hard-surface launch can accommodate trailer launches and has, according to the DEC, room to fit 55 vehicles. Navigating from the launch site to Janacks Landing should not be too difficult if you follow the western shore into Dead Creek Flow Bay.

DIRECTIONS: Turn onto CR 61/Main Street from NY 3, 6 miles east of Star Lake and 8 miles west of Cranberry Lake. Bear right at 0.8 miles onto Main Street, and continue over the steel bridge crossing the Oswegatchie River. The parking area is the one past the intersection on your right.

GPS Trailhead Coordinates	28 Cat Mountain
UTM Zone (WGS 84):	18T
Easting:	0506159.4
Northing:	4886517.1
Latitude:	N 44° 07' 54.56"
Longitude:	W 74° 55' 22.81"

29 Floodwood

SCENERY: ✿ ✿ ✿ ✿	SOLITUDE: ✿ ✿ ✿ ✿
TRAIL CONDITION: ✿ ✿ ✿	DISTANCE: *8.5 miles*
CHILDREN: ✿ ✿ ✿	HIKING TIME: *3–4 hours*
DIFFICULTY: ✿ ✿ ✿	OUTSTANDING FEATURES: *Multiple ponds*

At first glance, this hike may seem long, but the gently rolling terrain makes it an easy and relatively quick hike. Winding through a hardwood forest, the trail leads you from one pristine pond to another, offering excellent scenery and solitude the whole trip. Though the trail starts and ends in a bustling campground, it is likely that the only people you will encounter are canoeists at the numerous portages that crisscross the trail.

🚶 The trailhead is slightly different from the other Adirondack trailheads in that, first, access is through a campground, which includes a day-use fee of $8; second, no designated parking is located immediately nearby; and last, there is no trail register. The fee is waived if you are camping at either Fish Creek Pond or Rollins Pond campgrounds; for a description of the latter, see *The Best of Tent Camping: New York State*. The parking areas closest to the trailhead are in the day-use area near the swimming beach (go left after the registration booth) or near the basketball courts and recreation area, past the boat launch area, near campsite 50 (go right after the registration booth). Make sure that you grab a campground map, as it makes finding the trailhead easier and includes a trail map. The trailhead is located on the access road for Fish Creek Pond campsites C1 through C7. While walking up the road, you will see red DEC snowmobile trail markers and will come upon two log stumps that act as vehicle barriers on your right. You can begin here or farther up the road near campsite C7. The trail description included here is from the vehicle barrier heading north along the eastern leg and returning southward along the western leg. There is little difference heading clockwise or counterclockwise, though if you plan to walk only

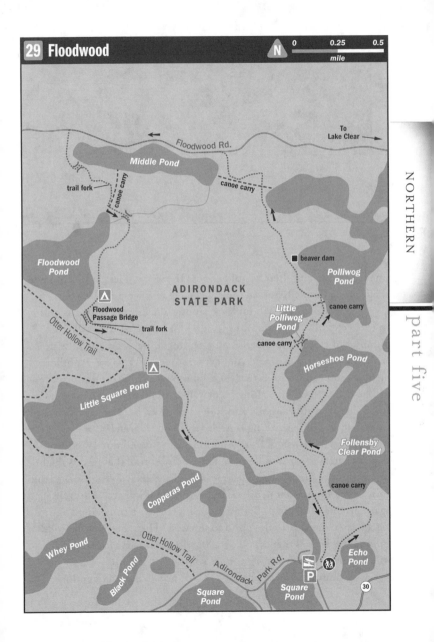

To
Lake Clear

Floodwood Rd.

Middle Pond

trail fork

canoe carry

canoe carry

beaver dam

Floodwood
Pond

ADIRONDACK
STATE PARK

Polliwog
Pond

canoe carry

Floodwood
Passage Bridge

Little
Polliwog
Pond

trail fork

canoe carry

Otter Hollow Trail

canoe carry

Horseshoe Pond

Little Square Pond

Follensby
Clear Pond

canoe carry

Copperas Pond

Otter Hollow Trail

Whey Pond

Adirondack Park Rd.

Echo
Pond

Black Pond

Square
Pond

Square
Pond

P

30

one leg of the trip, then I would choose the western leg, as it is in better shape and a flooded area on the eastern leg may seem impassable.

The trail winds north under a canopy of tall pines as well as multiple species of birch, and within a few hundred yards you will catch glimpses of Echo Pond. Dense pine saplings quickly dampen the noise from the campground, and you feel removed and remote. Another element you will notice is that the trail is basically flat, and your pace will be closer to walking along a sidewalk than hiking. Trail markers switch between snowmobile and foot-trail disks, but the path is so distinct that very little marking is necessary. You will catch glimpses of the much larger Follensby Clear Pond to your right and quickly come to a distinct intersection at mile 0.7. The east-west trail that bisects the hiking trail is the first of several canoe carries and provides a portage from Fish Creek Pond to Follensby Clear Pond. You will cross this portage again on the return trip, but for now, it provides a convenient way to get an up-close view of the pond to the west. The more heavily trodden canoe carry reveals that canoeing is the dominant activity in the area, which provides the hiker a bit more solitude on the trail.

Continuing straight ahead, you will notice that the hemlocks

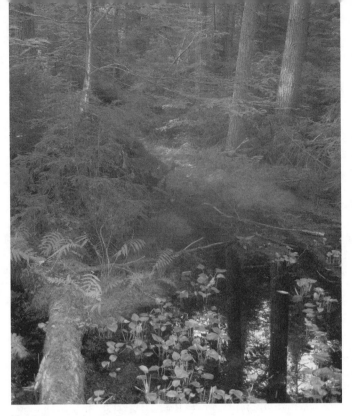

Flooded section along trail

and birches are quite large and tower overhead. Deep views into the forest contrast with limited views out onto the bodies of water, as hemlock saplings crowd the shorelines. At 1 mile, you first encounter Horseshoe Pond and walk along its edge through thicker hemlocks. At 1.4 miles, you come to a large moss-covered, mucky area that is the beginning of a spruce swamp bisected by the trail. At 1.8 miles, it may seem like you are coming up on another pond, but it is the opposite leg of Horseshoe Pond. The shore is distinctly more visible to your right as you head more directly north. At 2.3 miles, you come to the outlet of Little Polliwog Pond as it empties into Horseshoe Pond. A sign warns that the bridge is out; indeed, the bridge has fallen apart, though remnants of rickety boards laid on logs provide a zigzag crossing. On the other side, the trail briefly shares the canoe carry between Little Polliwog and Horseshoe ponds. At mile 2.9, you come across the canoe carry between Little Polliwog and Polliwog ponds through a stand of hemlocks.

Around 3 miles, you arrive at a broad, flooded section of the trail created by a recently constructed beaver dam. At this point your options for crossing the flooded section are limited. Crossing on top of the dam will likely be your driest option, but don't count on having dry feet afterward. The trail on the other side is less clear and is overgrown, and trail markers seemed to be missing when I was there. However, though the trail appears to be more of a herd path, it does continue through a couple of muddy areas, and red trail markers are visible again in less than 0.3 miles. You pass by another bay of Polliwog Pond at 3.2 miles, and at 3.4 miles, you come to a T in the path. Signs indicate that the snowmobile trail continues to your left. The path joining the trail from your right is the canoe carry between Polliwog Pond and Middle Pond. Head west (to your left) along the combined trail and portage for less than 0.3 miles, where the portage continues straight ahead and the trail veers to the right toward Floodwood Road. Less than 0.1 mile ahead is Floodwood Road, which you will follow 1 mile westward to pick up the western leg of the loop. It might seem odd to include a road with a trail, but the road is actually a pleasant variation on the trip. This seldom-used dirt road passes within feet of Middle Pond, and because it is free of roots and other obstructions, you can spend the mile looking out on the placid waters of the pond. You will pass one of several designated primitive campsites along the road.

At 4.7 miles, you pick the trail up again and head back into the woods along a ridge that sits above Middle Pond. In less than 0.3 miles, the trail heads east and you cross a log bridge. You will

Follensby Clear Pond

have left the shores of Middle Pond by now, but you have another chance to return to its shores at 5.1 miles, when you arrive at a fork in the trail. Continuing south along the trail, you catch glimpses of Floodwood Pond just before you reach yet another fork; the path ahead leads to the pond's shores, while the trail continues on your left. Pallets laid in pairs form a bridge across a stream, the outlet of Middle Pond into Floodwood Pond, at 5.4 miles. Shortly after the crossing, you come back to Floodwood Pond and stroll along its shores for the next 0.5 miles. At 6 miles, you pass through a designated campsite near where Floodwood Pond flows into a creek. Take a left at the campsite, and head west for 0.1 mile, where you reach another fork in the trail. To the right are Floodwood Passage Bridge and Otter Hollow Trail; these take you back to the campgrounds, while Floodwood Trail continues straight ahead beside the creek. Follow Floodwood Trail as it climbs slightly alongside the creek and then descends around 6.5 miles to another designated campsite. These designated campsites are used by canoeists and kayakers, but if they are vacant, their picnic tables make an excellent spot to stop, sit, and enjoy the scenery. The trail turns to your left at the campsite and continues along the shore of Little Square Pond through a couple more designated campsites.

The trail continues southeasterly along Little Square Pond as it transitions into Fish Creek Pond. From this point on, the trail delves deeper into the forest, and views of the water are limited to occasional glimpses. At mile 8, you pass the first canoe carry you encountered near the beginning and quickly come to the end of the trail at campsite C7.

DIRECTIONS: From Tupper Lake, head east on NY 3/NY 30. At 5.3 miles, turn left to stay on NY 30. At 5.4 miles, turn left at the main entrance to the Fish Creek Pond and Rollins Pond campgrounds. You will have to pay a day-use fee of $8, unless you are camping at either campground. The main parking area is to the left of the registration booth. The trailhead is along the access road to campsites C1 through C7.

GPS Trailhead Coordinates	29 Floodwood
UTM Zone (WGS 84):	18T
Easting:	0551111.5
Northing:	4906313.1
Latitude:	N 44° 18' 29.80"
Longitude:	W 74° 21' 33.00"

30 High Falls

SCENERY: ✿ ✿ ✿ ✿	DISTANCE: *16.2 miles*
TRAIL CONDITION: ✿ ✿ ✿ ✿	HIKING TIME: *Overnight*
CHILDREN: ✿ ✿	OUTSTANDING FEATURES: *Isolated waterfall,*
DIFFICULTY: ✿ ✿	*numerous beaver dams, wetlands and ponds, winding-*
SOLITUDE: ✿ ✿ ✿ ✿ ✿	*flat river, lakeside hiking, excellent berry picking*

With a wide variety of habitats and mostly easy trekking, this is an excellent introductory backpacking trip. Beaver activity is practically everywhere, with several dam tops forming part of the trail, so don't expect to keep your feet dry for long. In midsummer, the abundance of blueberries turns foraging practically into hike-by food service.

🚶🚶 Parking is available on either end of the loop and roughly 0.5 miles of road in between. Hikers will have to make the roadside trek either before or after their wilderness experience. With merely 0.5 miles and limited parking in each area, the use of two cars seems extravagant. My recommendation is for backpackers to stow their packs at the trailhead on which they wish to start, park at the other trailhead, and walk back to their desired start. You can hike the trail in either direction: Heading counterclockwise, High Falls is 9 miles; heading clockwise, it is 6.5 miles. A side trip to Cat Mountain (described on page 192) can be added to the clockwise approach or on the return, making the mileage on the eastern leg the same. I recommend that you camp at High Falls, but if time or weather forces you to camp early, designated riverside campsites (briefly described below) are located along the western leg, while camping along the eastern leg will require short bushwhacks to adhere to DEC wilderness camping regulations. Trail directions below are heading counterclockwise.

From the western parking area, walk around the tennis court down the private road to a vehicle barrier gate just past a residence on your right. The trail register is a little beyond the barrier and

N

0   0.75   1.5

miles

To
Cranberry

3

3

Inlet Rd.

Ranger School Rd.

CR 61

South Shore Rd.

Dead Creek Flow

Oswegatchie River

Skate Creek

P

P

**ADIRONDACK
STATE PARK**

**FIVE PONDS
WILDERNESS**

Janacks
Landing

side trip
to Cat Mountain

Cat
Mountain

Dead Creek

Oswegatchie River

**High Rock Trail
intersection**

Glasby
Pond

Cowhorn
Junction Trail

Cat
Mountain
Pond

Bassout
Pond

**Roundtop
Mountain**

Glasby Creek

Sand Hill Trail

**Threemile
Mountain**

Oswegatchie River

old machinery

lean-to

High Falls

Oswegatchie River

Nicks
Pond

Buck Brook

Wolf Pond Outlet

Big
Five

**Panther
Mountain**

**Partlow
Mountain**

Robinson River

**Greenfield
Mountain**

has a map of the area, including 46 designated campsites along the Oswegatchie River. Most of these sites are either across the river or require bushwhacking, so these are mainly used by canoeists and kayakers. The first mile of the trail is along a grass-covered gravel road, which provides access for municipal water. With the trail free of any obstructions, you will have the opportunity to look out for wildlife in the dammed section of Skate Creek on your left. A little more than 0.5 miles in, you will cross Skate Creek, and its wetland will sprawl off to your right. These broad, marshy areas are very common in the northern section of the Adirondacks and are often seen from the road but are not frequently traversable on foot. Approximately 1 mile in, the trail crosses a stream that feeds into Skate Creek and begins to climb as you plunge into a mixed hardwood forest. It would be hard to get lost along this wide-open road, but red DEC markers provide reassurance that you are headed in the right direction. At 1.8 miles, you will come to a clearing where an overgrown road climbs to your left. In the past, numerous roads and paths headed more directly to the High Falls area, but the microburst windstorm of 1995 created so much blowdown that these trails have been abandoned. Beyond the

One of the many flooded areas due to the abundance of beaver activity in the area

clearing, ferns and other deciduous plants encroach on the trail, but
its past use as a road is unmistakable, as it is broad, flat, free of
typical obstructions, and elevated above the surrounding terrain. The
western half of the trail is almost entirely composed of abandoned
roads, which makes its 9 miles nearly equivalent in effort to the
6.5-mile hike along the eastern leg. At 2.3 miles, the canopy opens,
and another creek with a broad wetland sprawls out on your right.
Despite being flanked by short evergreens, the trail is open to the sky.
At this point, you have reached the plateau that the western leg traverses, and the rest of the way gently rolls along at this elevation. During the summer, the trailside will be thick with highbush blueberries.
At 3.8 miles, you will reenter the hardwood forest and come to a fork

in the trail. A tenth of a mile to your right is High Rock, which over-looks the Oswegatchie River. The boulder that provides an outlook across the meandering river is actually not very high. However, the plain through which the river cuts its veritable maze is so broad that you can see quite far. A popular campsite is also located here, so do not be surprised to see your first group of boaters. Though the Oswegatchie flows north to the west of the trail, this side trip will be your only opportunity to see it for several miles.

Heading south, you walk over a stone-and-concrete bridge that spans a stream at 4.3 miles. At 5.3 miles, you encounter the first of many beaver dams that have created wide marshlands both up- and downstream. To cross this and future dammed sections, you will walk along the tops of the dams. Picking your way atop the dams is not difficult, but wet feet are inevitable. Aside from the wet areas created by the beaver dams, the trail is relatively level and easygoing along these old logging roads. Less than 1 mile ahead, mile 6.1, you traverse another dammed section, and then shortly after, reenter the forest. A half mile later, the trail meets the Oswegatchie, as well as the first of three easily accessible designated campsites along the river. The first site, with no number, is directly on the trail, while a short way ahead, a path leads to site 28, which is masked from the trail by a stand of thick saplings. This site also has the advantage of sitting just above a small flume that adds interest to the mostly flat river. Shortly after this brief encounter with the river, you head back into wetland territory along another stream and then back into the forest, where you reach a fork in the trail, 7.5 miles. Trail signs indicate that High Falls is 1.5 miles ahead, while the fork to the right takes you deep into the Five Ponds Wilderness. Shortly ahead, you enter an area where Glasby Creek and the Oswegatchie River meet. This confluence creates a broad wetland and meadow setting with beaver activity throughout. Yellow disks indicate a couple of designated campsites in the area, but their locations escaped me. Many of the designated campsites either were affected by the 1995 microburst storm or see little use because most people are headed to the High Falls lean-tos or campsites. After crossing a log-and-plank bridge, the trail climbs through a short section of stunted pines that gradually gives way to mixed hardwoods.

At mile 8.6, you reach an intersection; High Falls is 0.5 miles to the right, while it is 6.1 miles back to Wanakena along the eastern leg. Along the trail to High Falls, you will come upon an abandoned and heavily rusted piece of machinery. Its presence adds a quaint reminder that, not too long ago, this area was used by industry, but the wilderness quickly reestablishes itself and wipes out all but the most persistent traces of human activity. After a brief climb, you will hear High Falls and then come to designated campsite 16 and the confluence of several paths, 9.1 miles. The trail directly to the right is the canoe carry that bypasses the falls. A path slightly to your right leads to a boulder at the base of the falls. A path to the left leads to one of the pit toilets in the area. The path straight ahead leads to the start of the canoe carry, the top of the falls, and the lean-to on this side of the river. The falls are only 20 feet tall but are still excellent. The water bifurcates, forming a spray on the left and a rushing torrent on the right. The pool at the base is deep enough to swim in, and while I was there, a heron fishing for brown trout occupied it.

The return trip along the eastern leg is a sharp contrast to the easy hiking along the old logging roads of the western leg. However, it is no different from typical trails in the Adirondacks, except perhaps for the vast amount of beaver activity. Following blue DEC disks, head east from the junction with the western leg; total mileage before starting this leg is 9.6 miles. After picking your way up and over a hillock, where damage from the 1995 microburst storm is still evident, you reach a broad wetland in less than 0.5 miles. A large fallen pine tree forms a bridge over the stream here, which should be carefully negotiated, especially when wet. The next 2.2 miles take you along the base of Threemile Mountain through myriad wetlands created by successive beaver dams. The mix of forest and open marshlands created by the beaver dams creates some very interesting scenery complemented by the

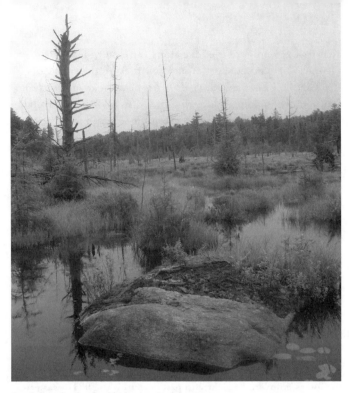

Another wetland created by beavers in the area

abundance of berry-picking opportunities, including blueberry, raspberry, black caps, and blackberries, depending on the season.

At 12.2 miles, you reach the intersection of the eastern leg with Cowhorn Junction Trail on the right. This intersection is Sand Hill Junction, where a side trip up to Cat Mountain is highly recommended. Red DEC disks now mark the trail, and you will be heading generally north as the trail begins to descend. You will have to negotiate a few more wet areas before reaching a trail register at the intersection with Janacks Landing Trail. Less than 0.3 miles to the right is a lean-to and boat landing for hikers who wish to boat in and avoid the initial 2.8 miles of the hike along the eastern leg. The nearest boat launch is 7.8 miles away, as the crow flies, in the village of Cranberry Lake; the boat launch is off NY 3 near the dam. Most of the remaining hike is along old logging roads, so hiking in is likely the fastest and most direct approach. From the intersection, the trail veers west for 0.5 miles, where it crosses Dead Creek. Dead Creek Flow is the largest submerged bay of Cranberry Lake. The distinction may sound peculiar until you realize that this bay was previously the creek bed until Cranberry Lake was dammed in 1867. The hike around the western point of Dead Creek Flow adds yet another scenic element. After coming around the western point, you reach a large designated campground and the beginning of the old logging road, which will take you back to Wanakena. The road climbs with a gentle grade, and you will encounter a few more beaver-flooded areas before reaching the eastern trail at 16.2 miles.

DIRECTIONS: Turn onto County Road 61/Main Street from NY 3, 6 miles east of Star Lake and 8 miles west of Cranberry Lake. Bear right at 0.8 miles onto Main Street, and continue over the steel bridge crossing the Oswegatchie River. The closest parking area is approximately 0.5 miles past the intersection on the right, just past the tennis court. The eastern parking lot is another 0.5 miles on the right.

GPS Trailhead Coordinates	30 High Falls
UTM Zone (WGS 84):	18T
Easting:	0506159.4
Northing:	4886517.1
Latitude:	N 44° 07' 54.56"
Longitude:	W 74° 55' 22.81"

SCENERY: ✿ ✿ ✿ ✿	DISTANCE: *1 mile round-trip to falls, 3 miles*
TRAIL CONDITION: ✿ ✿ ✿ ✿	*along river*
CHILDREN: ✿ ✿ ✿ ✿ ✿	HIKING TIME: *1–2 hours*
DIFFICULTY: ✿	OUTSTANDING FEATURES: *Waterfall,*
SOLITUDE: ✿ ✿	*riverside walk*

As one of a few hikes with sections that are wheelchair accessible, this trail is ideal for families with limited mobility or who just prefer a trip that does not require constant weaving around obstacles. If you prefer obstacles, you can always extend your trip to include the riverside trail and a little extra bushwhacking downstream to explore some interesting cataracts and flumes. Lampson Falls is also a popular swimming spot during the summer, but if you continue along the riverside trail, you will find solitude.

🚶🚶 Parking for the trailhead is parallel to County Road 27; two of the five designated spaces are reserved for handicapped parking, though an additional car or two could fit in behind the regular parking spaces. The trail begins at the southern end of the pullout, past a vehicle barrier. The trail is actually a crushed-gravel access road, which is why it is designated universally accessible. The trail register and a map of the trail system are located a little less than 0.3 miles past the vehicle barrier. The forest is a mixture of eastern white pines and hardwoods with a lush and thick understory of ferns. The terrain, befitting an accessible trail, is exceptionally flat, and you will hear the roar of the falls long before you reach the accessible viewing area. Follow the wide path through a series of switchbacks and numerous turning points, constructed out of landscape timbers and filled with gravel, to the viewing spot above the falls. From the top of the falls, it is easy to see why this is a popular attraction, as the whole of Grass River cascades down over the exposed bedrock in a frothy torrent. From this vantage point, keep an eye out for the swifts that swoop and dive as they ride updrafts and feast

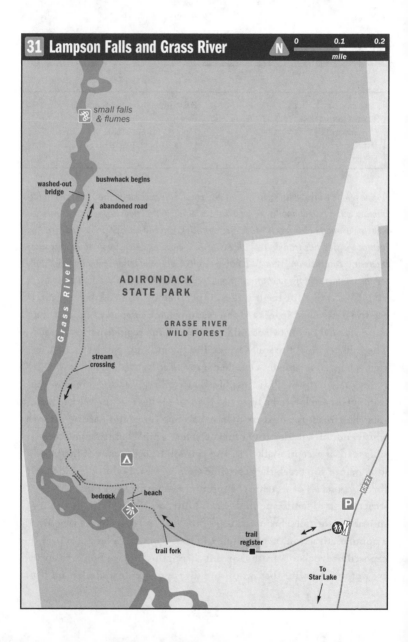

N

0   0.1   0.2
mile

small falls
& flumes

washed-out
bridge

bushwhack begins

abandoned road

Grass River

**ADIRONDACK
STATE PARK**

**GRASSE RIVER
WILD FOREST**

stream
crossing

CR 27

P

bedrock

beach

trail fork

trail
register

To
Star Lake

on insects caught above the falls. To reach the base of the falls, you can choose any number of footpaths or scramble down the rocks, but the accessible portion of the trail ends here.

At the base of the falls is a sandy beach that is an obvious congregation point and an unfortunate reminder that not all people follow the DEC's carry-in, carry-out policy. This is an easy place to implement one of my preferred policies: Carry in, carry one more out. From the sandy beach, you can scramble up a steep hillside to reach exposed portions of bedrock directly across from the waterfall. This is my favorite vantage point of the falls and is an excellent spot to stop and enjoy the view. Back among the tall pines is a designated camping area that includes the standard pit toilet but offers no views of the waterfall or river. Continue along the bedrock, across from the falls, to a rocky peninsula for another excellent picnicking spot, as well as the beginning of the riverside trail.

At the time of this writing, the trail was in serious disrepair, with multiple areas of nearly impassable blowdown. However, DEC and volunteer trail crews clear blowdown regularly, so the trail may have been returned to a suitable condition, making it an easy riverside

Frothy cataract downstream of the trail's end

stroll. Otherwise, be prepared to undertake some three-dimensional limbo as you contort your way through the barricades of downed trees. Marked with red disks, the trail is evidently rarely used, and thick overgrown vegetation on either side masks the conditions underfoot. Brambles are a significant part of the overgrowth, so gaiters are recommended during the summer. Additionally numerous beaver plunge holes are hidden by the dense overgrowth, so use caution when you cannot see your footing.

In sharp contrast to the turbulent falls, the river seems almost placid, and its grass- and fern-lined banks make for a tranquil setting. At 1.5 miles, the trail intersects an overgrown road to your right, and the remnants of a foundation are visible on both banks. Readers of the old trail guides will discover that the bridge connecting the two banks was washed out in 1998 and has not been replaced. The foundations sit on either side of a small flume, where the river narrows from dozens of feet to just a few feet. This is the formal end of the trail, which is unfortunate because several flumes, falls, and cataracts farther downstream add great interest to the trip. To see these spectacles, you will have to follow old footpaths and bushwhack a bit, but rest assured, other hikers have been here before, so the path is distinct most of the way. Over the next 0.3 miles, the placid waters transform into frothing cascades, as the river drops quickly and the lush, wide banks constrict to rocky ledges. You will see multiple flumes and falls along the paths, but my favorite is where the river forks at a tiny rocky island. The eastern fork drops vertically to form a narrow waterfall, after which the flow diminishes into slack water, while the western leg forms a frothing cataract. The island can be reached by crossing above the tiny waterfall or rock-hopping in the slack water. This section of the river coincides with the disappearance of the old footpaths and makes a good end for the river exploration.

DIRECTIONS: From Star Lake, head northwest along NY 3, and turn right onto CR 27/CR 27-A. Continue 0.8 miles and turn right onto CR 27 heading north. Follow CR 27 north 8.1 miles, and turn right to stay on CR 27. Continue on CR 27 another 4.2 miles, passing the airstrip along the way. The parking area will be on your left.

GPS Trailhead Coordinates	31 Lampson Falls and Grass River
UTM Zone (WGS 84):	18T
Easting:	0495115.6
Northing:	4916862.3
Latitude:	N 44° 24' 18.12"
Longitude:	W 75° 03' 40.83"

32 Owls Head Mountain

SCENERY: ☆ ☆ ☆ ☆	DISTANCE: *6.3 miles*
TRAIL CONDITION: ☆ ☆ ☆ ☆	HIKING TIME: *3–4 hours*
CHILDREN: ☆ ☆ ☆ ☆ ☆	OUTSTANDING FEATURES: *Panoramic views,*
DIFFICULTY: ☆	*fire tower, historic site*
SOLITUDE: ☆ ☆ ☆	

On the boundary of the West–Central and Northern sections of the Adirondacks is the scenic peak Owls Head. By climbing the accessible fire tower on the summit, you have a 360-degree view of the surrounding hills and lakes. The remains of an old observer cabin add some historical interest as well.

🏃 The trailhead and register are located on the left side of the small parking pullout. The parking area is located on a curve along Endion Road and may accommodate a dozen cars if visitors park thoughtfully. The trail, marked with red disks, immediately begins to ascend amid a dense maple and beech hardwood forest. After 0.3 miles, the trail levels off and follows mostly rolling terrain for another 1.3 miles. At 1 mile from the trailhead, you reach an intersection with another trail. To your left is the trail to Owls Head summit, 2.1 miles away, while to your right is a trail to NY 30, 3.5 miles, and Lake Eaton Campground, 3.8 miles. Shortly after the first intersection, you pass an abandoned foot trail on your right, followed by an old road that joins the main trail from behind. The old road has orange placards with white diamonds on them. A few of these placards, as well as snowmobile disks, are interspersed with the red DEC trail markers along the main trail. Aside from the previously mentioned intersections, the trail runs in a relatively straight southwest direction to the summit and is easy to follow.

At 2 miles, the trail swings south and begins to ascend gradually and then more steeply at 2.3 miles. A seasonal stream flows on your

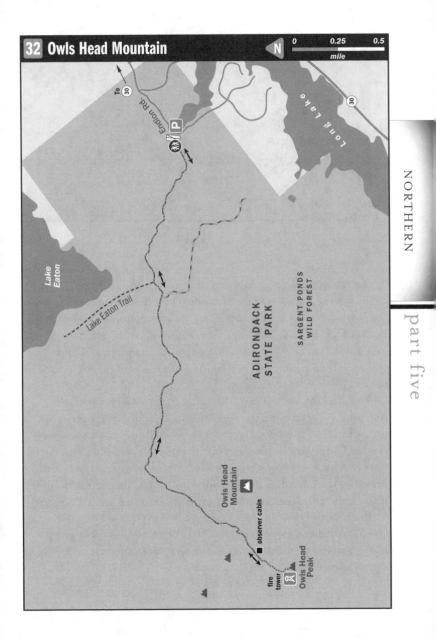

N

0   0.25   0.5
mile

Long Lake

To 30

Endion Rd.

P

Lake Eaton

Lake Eaton Trail

ADIRONDACK
STATE PARK

SARGENT PONDS
WILD FOREST

Owls Head
Mountain

■ observer cabin

fire
tower

Owls Head Peak

NORTHERN

part five

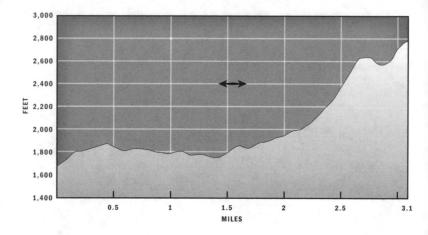

left as you climb through sections of heavy erosion. You reach a crest in the trail at 2.7 miles. You have not yet reached the summit but are passing between two points along the mountain that resemble the horns of an owl. The trail dips down, less than 100 feet of elevation, into a small valley before climbing steeply to the summit. Before you make the final ascent, you pass by the former site of the cabin used by the fire tower's observer.

Around the turn of the 20th century, forest fires swept the Adirondack region, and nearly 1 million acres of forest burned throughout the preserve. In response to this destruction, the state erected fire towers atop many peaks throughout the Adirondacks. The tasks of state-employed observers included locating and triangulating fires. On the side, they also provided innumerable hikers with information and conservation education. A wooden fire tower was erected on the peak of Owls Head around 1911. It was replaced by a steel tower in 1919 and closed in 1979. After restoration work was complete, it was reopened in 2004, and efforts are currently underway to continue maintenance of the tower.

The final climb to the summit passes over exposed portions of ledge and includes multiple small switchbacks. You will need to use both hands in several sections. The trail suddenly ends as you come through a thick stand of firs near the base of the steel fire tower. Multiple grassy patches threaded through the exposed portions of the summit (elevation: 2,812 feet) make excellent picnic areas. A large slab of exposed rock juts out to the southwest, providing an outstanding lookout. For a 360-degree view of the area, you should climb the fire tower. The fence-enclosed stairs lead to a wooden platform covered by a steel cap typical of the fire towers that are still in use in the Adirondacks.

Perhaps on your way up you noticed old utility poles along the sides of the trail. If not, they are more noticeable on your way back down. The two opposing "branches" on these poles also resemble owls' horns, making the name of this trail doubly apt.

DIRECTIONS: From the north intersection of NY 30 and NY 28 N in Long Lake, head northwest on NY 30. Turn left onto Endion Road, 1.3 miles. Follow Endion Road 1.6 miles, and look for the gravel pullout on the right.

GPS Trailhead Coordinates	32 Owls Head Mountain
UTM Zone (WGS 84):	18T
Easting:	0543891.8
Northing:	4867968.3
Latitude:	N 43° 57' 48.73"
Longitude:	W 74° 27' 10.37"

33 Saint Regis Mountain

SCENERY: ✸ ✸ ✸ ✸	DISTANCE: *6.7 miles*
TRAIL CONDITION: ✸ ✸ ✸ ✸	HIKING TIME: *3–4 hours*
CHILDREN: ✸ ✸ ✸	OUTSTANDING FEATURES: *Panoramic views,*
DIFFICULTY: ✸ ✸ ✸	*fire tower*
SOLITUDE: ✸ ✸	

Best known for its mostly flat terrain, the northern section of the Adirondacks has many excellent extended canoe trips. Most notable is the Saint Regis Canoe Area. However, looming over this area of hundreds of ponds, lakes, and interconnected waterways is St. Regis Mountain. For a truly majestic view, the namesake summit cannot be surpassed.

🏃 The actual trailhead is a short distance south of the large and well-maintained parking area. From the parking area, no signs point you to the trail. To reach the trail, head south down Topridge Road across the Saint Regis River, whose rushing waters you probably noticed as soon as you parked. Approximately 0.1 mile down the road, you will see the trail register just off to your right. Next to the register is a finely built log-and-plank bridge that is indicative of ongoing work to maintain the trail. Indeed, the presence of so many mucky areas, despite the amount of maintenance, shows how popular this trail is. The DEC constructed the bridge when it rerouted the trail, but forestry students from Paul Smith's College and stewards have done much of the work evident throughout. Anyone wishing for solitude atop the mountain would be wise to follow a few rules of thumb. First, hike during the week rather than on weekends, and especially avoid holiday weekends. Second, hike when school is in session. Last, start earlier, which usually ensures you some time to yourself at the peak and other destinations where hikers typically congregate.

Following the red disks that mark the trail, you will be hiking a generally rolling terrain through mature hardwoods dotted with large hemlocks. Approximately 0.3 miles in, you will pass a sheer rock face covered in moss and ferns. This adds some variation to the hike, but the dominant feature before reaching the summit is the deep forest. At I mile, you will walk over a small hillock heavily shaded by hemlocks and then descend briefly back into the mixed hardwood forest. The trail becomes very straight and begins to climb afterward, but the grade is gradual and almost difficult to notice. You pass an orange painted pipe surrounded by stones on the left at 1.7 miles; this is approximately the halfway point of the trail. After a slight descent around mile 2.1, you come to a fork in the trail and a bridge that crosses a small stream. The trail to your left is the old trail that is no longer maintained. Once you cross the bridge, the ascent to the summit truly begins. Gradual at first, it becomes much steeper as you near the summit. The stream you crossed flows on your right as you climb and occasionally flows over the trail nearer the summit. Stone steps built along the trail help prevent further erosion, but long sections of muddy areas become inevitable. Indeed, the trail has been

Spectacular view atop the summit

worn into a rut more than a foot deep. Estimating how far along these mires are is futile, as one slick seems to grow larger than the previous one, and you quickly lose track of how many you cross. At 2.9 miles, you pass a vertical rock face almost entirely covered in moss. Another distinct landmark is at mile 3.1, where you pass a large balancing rock on your left and another boulder directly to your right. Passage between these boulders is essentially the last portion of steep climbing, and the final elevation gains are over flatter portions. Winding around the contours of the peak, the trail is shaded by mostly paper birches with an occasional mountain ash. Keep an eye out on your right for a lookout, which offers good panoramic views and a glimpse of the fire tower.

Flat portion of the trail

At the summit, you have 360-degree views of the myriad lakes and ponds nestled among forested hills and small mountains within the immediate vicinity, with the High Peaks towering off to the south. The bottom stairs to the fire tower have been removed to prevent people from climbing, but its presence adds an interesting feature nonetheless. Its location in a canoe area is a much-debated issue. The DEC Master Plan calls for the removal of fire towers from wild forest areas, which include canoe areas, but revisions and conflicts with the New York Historic Preservation Act of 1980 complicate the matter. Many groups have formed to protect and restore fire towers on this and other peaks, claiming that fire towers are part of the region's history and that their stewards were instrumental in educating the public, helping to protect and preserve the wilderness. The tower's removal is on hold while these issues are resolved.

DIRECTIONS: From Tupper Lake, head east on NY 3/NY 30. Turn left to stay on NY 30 at 5.3 miles. At 14.3 miles, turn left again to stay on NY 30. Turn left on Keese Mill Road at 6.9 miles. The DEC parking area is 2.6 miles ahead on the left.

GPS Trailhead Coordinates	33 Saint Regis Mountain
UTM Zone (WGS 84):	18T
Easting:	0555780.4
Northing:	4919921.2
Latitude:	N 44° 25' 49.57"
Longitude:	W 74° 17' 57.02"

High Peaks Hikes (34-40)

N

0   5   10
miles

6

PART SIX
High Peaks Hikes

34 Ampersand Mountain

SCENERY: ✿ ✿ ✿ ✿
TRAIL CONDITION: ✿ ✿ ✿
CHILDREN: ✿ ✿
DIFFICULTY: ✿ ✿ ✿ ✿
SOLITUDE: ✿

DISTANCE: *5.2 miles*
HIKING TIME: *3–4 hours*
OUTSTANDING FEATURES: *Bald summit, panoramic views*

Ampersand Mountain sits on the confluence of the flat north and High Peaks regions of the Adirondacks. An extremely popular hike, it offers a varied experience as you transition from a gentle walk through tall hemlocks to a steep ascent over boulder stairs. Passage through enormous craggy boulders takes you to the bald summit, from which the lake sprawls out beneath you to the north and the High Peaks can be seen in the distance to the south.

When I approached on a sunny Saturday afternoon, it was clear that this trail is extremely popular. Dozens of cars lined NY 3 on both sides, and I could see that the small parking area was nowhere near adequate. While the lot also provides access to a short trail to Dutton Brook, the vast majority of hikers were climbing Ampersand Mountain. Indeed the trail register had been filled days before by the dozens of parties that hike the trail each day during the peak of summer. As with all popular trails, it is best to visit these in the off-season, during the week, or early if you have any desire for privacy.

Why is the trail so popular? It is likely that the combination of the easy stroll at the beginning through towering old-growth forest, its proximity to a major road and tourist destinations, and the spectacular views all contribute to its appeal. Unfortunately I reached the summit when a major thunderstorm had rolled in and visibility had dropped to several feet, so I cannot attest to the latter. Quite literally the peak was awash in a sheet of flowing rain, and I was stuck in a cloud. Lightning flashed in all directions, and fierce winds threatened to blow others and

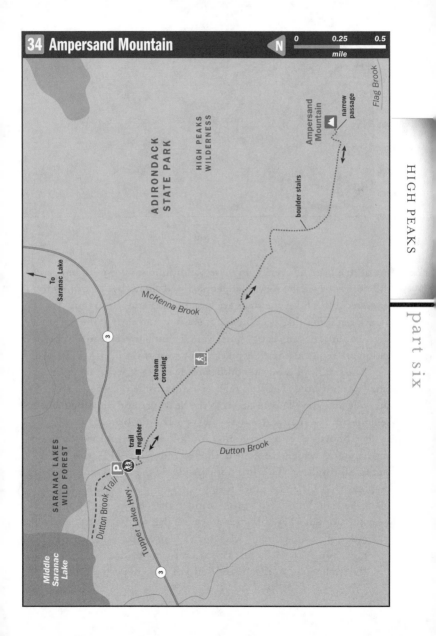

N

0   0.25   0.5
mile

Flag Brook

Ampersand Mountain

narrow passage

boulder stairs

HIGH PEAKS WILDERNESS

ADIRONDACK STATE PARK

McKenna Brook

To Saranac Lake

3

stream crossing

trail register

Dutton Brook

P

SARANAC LAKES WILD FOREST

Dutton Brook Trail

Tupper Lake Hwy.

3

Middle Saranac Lake

me off the peak. Lingering in these conditions was unwise at best, so I did not get to see the views that people raved about, but according to veterans of this hike, the views are breathtaking and panoramic. It was a stark reminder that even though it is sunny and clear at the start of a hike, conditions can change quickly, and a little precaution and preparation are required on every hike and in every season.

The trailhead is on the southern side of NY 3 across from the small parking area. The trail register is just inside the woods, and the wide and gravelly base attests to the heavy use and ongoing maintenance. In less than 0.3 miles, you cross Dutton Brook over a log bridge. Shortly after this crossing, you will definitely notice the towering hemlocks, which are some of the few remaining old-growth trees in the Adirondacks. This forest is considered the largest known sugar maple–yellow birch–hemlock forest in Adirondack Park. Red disks mark the trail, but it is so heavily trodden that, except for a few places near the summit where blowdown occurs, they are hardly necessary. At 0.8 miles, planks laid lengthwise form a boardwalk over a wet area. At 1 mile, you cross McKenna Brook over a log bridge. Past this crossing, the trail begins to climb, and you will rock-hop across streams

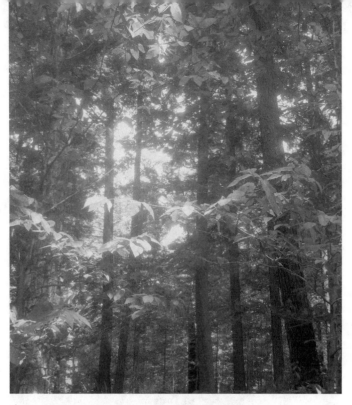

Tall hemlocks along the flat approach to the summit

and more mucky areas as the trail gradually becomes steep. The hemlocks that previously towered overhead give way to birches and maples, and the vast stonework employed to lessen the degree of erosion becomes evident. Long stretches of boulder stairs were constructed within the past decade to minimize the impact hikers had on the trail, once considered one of the most heavily eroded. Climbing only on the stone sections gives the forest a chance to regenerate some of its ground cover and, hopefully, forestalls further erosion. The last mile is basically a vertical climb and you need your hands free.

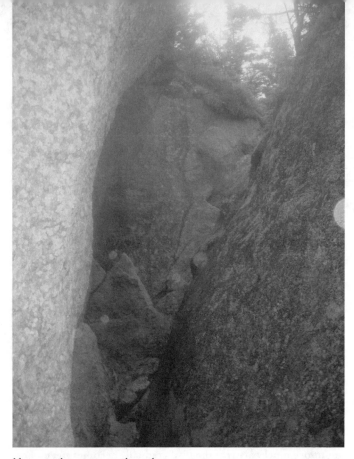

Narrow rock passage near the peak

As the forest transitions from hardwoods to stunted firs and
evergreens, the stonework diminishes until it becomes nonexistent,
and the erosion becomes severe. At this point, the various paths
chosen to bypass washed-out areas or precipitous sections make finding the trail difficult and the trail markers a necessity. Take your
time throughout the final climb, and use caution over eroded and

slippery surfaces. Around 2.3 miles, the trail levels off briefly just shy of the summit. You pass a few large boulders and eventually come to a passage between exposed faces of bedrock with a fissure opening up on your right. The trail then turns to your left and winds around to a rock face that you must scramble up and over. The roots of a tree will help you up, but after seeing the erosion caused by so many hikers, you can't help but wonder how much longer this tree will be around. Yellow arrows painted on the bald mountaintop point you in the direction of the easiest ways around the three knobs. Many of the bald peaks in the Adirondacks were created when Verplank Colvin burned the tops of mountains during his 19th-century survey of the region. Erosion soon swept away the topsoil, leaving the mountains bald. Each knob offers its own merits and vantage points, and curious hikers will also find the remnants of a fire tower as well as a plaque in memory of the Ampersand Hermit. The hermit, Walter Channing Rice, manned the fire tower from 1915 to 1923.

DIRECTIONS: From Tupper Lake, head east on NY 3/NY 30. At 5.3 miles, turn right to stay on NY 3. At 7.8 miles, the designated parking area is on your left. The parking area may be full, so take care when parking on the side of the road.

GPS Trailhead Coordinates	34 Ampersand Mountain
UTM Zone (WGS 84):	18T
Easting:	0560733.1
Northing:	4900069.5
Latitude:	N 44° 15' 4.62"
Longitude:	W 74° 14' 22.93"

35 Ausable River: *West River Trail*

SCENERY: ✿ ✿ ✿ ✿ ✿	DISTANCE: *5.4 miles one way*
TRAIL CONDITION: ✿ ✿ ✿ ✿ ✿	HIKING TIME: *3–4 hours one way*
CHILDREN: ✿ ✿ ✿	OUTSTANDING FEATURES: *Spectacular*
DIFFICULTY: ✿ ✿	*waterfalls, scenic lookout, riverside stroll*
SOLITUDE: ✿ ✿ ✿ ✿	

The East Branch of Ausable River is a smorgasbord of waterfalls. From mossy cascades and powerful flumes to misty veils and thunderous sheer drops, the variety and multitude of waterfalls make this an ideal waterfall lover's hike. The hike is rich with scenic lookouts and riverside strolling—overall an excellent excursion. Be advised, though, that it lies on private property (public access has been granted), so certain restrictions apply.

🕴🕴 The trail lies entirely within the property lines of the Adirondack Mountain Reserve (AMR), so hikers should be aware of several restrictions. The rules are strictly enforced and posted when entering the property. The main restrictions are that pets are not allowed, and no camping, hunting, fishing, swimming, or boating is allowed. Additionally, off-trail travel, bushwhacking, and rock climbing are prohibited. Despite the restrictions, one major advantage of the trail being on private property is its superb condition. There are few muddy areas, trails are clear of blowdown, and bridges are all in excellent condition. Parking (see directions below) is approximately 0.7 miles from the trailhead and register but is included in the mileage given.

The large parking area near NY 73 can accommodate dozens of cars, so finding a spot should be straightforward. Head west along Ausable Club Road. At a little more than 0.1 mile, you pass the trailhead for Round and Dix mountains. Roughly 0.3 miles later, you pass a second trailhead junction, Noonmark Trail, as well as a golf course. Just past the tennis courts, you will see a large lime-green building and reach Lake Road at 0.6 miles. Turn left down the road,

35 Ausable River: **West River Trail**

N

0   0.5   1
mile

Roaring Brook
Putnam Brook
Nubble
Roaring Brook Trail
73
Round Mountain
Round Pond Trail
N. Fork Bouquet River
Western Trail
DIX MOUNTAIN WILDERNESS
Dix Trail
Noonmark Mountain
Semson Trail
Ausable Club Rd.
P
To Keene
73
CR 86A
W. Branch Ausable River
AMR gate
Leach Trail
Dix Trail
ADIRONDACK STATE PARK
Ladies Mile Trail
Cathedral Rocks
Lake Rd.
Bear Den Mountain
Snow Mountain Trail
Deer Brook
Cathedral Rocks and Bear Run Trail
Wedge Brook Cascades
Artists Falls
Hedgehog Mountain
W. A. White Trail
waterfall lookout
Gill Brook
Indian Head Trail
W. A. White Trail
Wedge Brook Trail
Beaver Meadows Falls
Gill Brook Trail
Indian Head
HIGH PEAKS WILDERNESS
maintenance building
Indian Head Lookout
Lower Wolfjaw Mountain
Lower Wolf Trail
Beaver Meadows Trail
West River Trail
Lower Ausable Lake
Lost Lookout Trail
Rainbow Falls
ADR Range Trail
Upper Wolfjaw Mountain
trail fork to Gothics
trail fork to Sawteeth
A. E. Weld Trail
Armstrong Mountain
Scenic Trail

and head past several small cabins to the AMR trail register. All hikers must sign in and out at the register. Continue down the road past the ornate wooden gate. A gabled arch, constructed from round and irregular logs and branches, vaults the gate, which is constructed similarly and has AMR built into its center. The gate was reconstructed in 1986 as a part of the AMR's centennial observances and is a replica of the original.

Shortly after the gate, you pass Ladies Mile Trail, which, if you want to get off the club's road sooner, will also lead to West River Trail. A second intersection with Ladies Mile Trail is 0.3 miles past the gate, 1 mile total. This junction connects to West River Trail directly, but yards ahead is a junction with East River Trail (an alternate way to reach West River Trail) and likely your return trip if you make the complete loop. Cross the wooden plank bridge, and head 0.3 miles west to another trail junction. Straight ahead are East River Trail and the path back to Lake Road, while Bear Run, Cathedral Rocks, and West River trails are off to the right. Cross the bridge over the East Branch of Ausable River, and turn left onto the trail. West River Trail, marked with yellow markers,

Adirondack Mountain Reserve gates

heads west, while Bear Run and Cathedral Rocks trails, marked in red, head north.

The trail heads west under towering hemlocks and climbs gradually above the river gorge. At times you hike close to the river, but you veer away into the surrounding forest over many sections. Grades are gentle, and at 1.7 miles, you cross Pyramid Brook, after which the trail heads back toward the river. At 1.8 miles, you reconnect with Bear Run, Cathedral Rocks, and Pyramid Brook trails. Approximately 0.1 mile ahead, you reach another junction and a green trail sign indicating East River Trail, Lake Road, and Canyon Bridge to your left; West River Trail and Wolfjaw straight ahead; and Bear Run, Cathedral Rocks, and West River trails back the way you came. The trail climbs a bit past this intersection, and the drop down to the river is significant at this point. You can see small cascades and flumes along the river, and the roaring of the water drowns out most sounds. The sounds and views decrease as you climb away from the river for the next 0.5 miles, but you soon return; at 2.4 miles you come across a lookout to a waterfall along the river. This lookout is to the left of the trail, and there is a precipitous drop, so take care while viewing the waterfall. Shortly after, the trail swings northward to follow a feeder brook, Wedge Brook, a short distance and then crosses the brook over a bridge. The bridge spans the brook between two waterfalls. The lower is really a small cascade, and the second is a small waterfall that branches around a large rock and tumbles into a pool above the bridge. On the other side is Wedge Brook Trail to Lower Wolfjaw, and a sign indicates that the Wedge Brook Cascades are a couple hundred yards away. A short climb up this trail reveals a series of small cascades that weave their way down mossy crevices in the rock to the small pool below.

Back along the main trail, you reach the river in less than 0.3 miles, and you will notice that it is now surging through tight flumes and small cascades at many points. At 2.9 miles, you see another waterfall, which is approximately 25 feet high with a very powerful surge of water that spurts out nearly horizontally as the river is restricted a few feet through the narrow gorge. Occasional vantage points are available, but take care when trying to view this fall, as the river gorge is very steep and treacherous. After this waterfall, the river levels off and spreads out among the boulders, but many tiny falls and cascades remain throughout.

At 3.3 miles, the trail reaches a small brook and turns north almost immediately after you reach Beaver Meadow Falls. Unlike the last falls, which fell in a powerful surge, Beaver Meadow Falls is almost like a light rain or mist. Often referred to as a bridal-veil falls, Beaver Meadow Falls is about 60 feet high. A bridge that spans the brook provides an excellent place to admire and photograph the falls.

West River Trail continues along the river westward through some marshy sections and slow-flowing waters that add variety and interest. However, a side trip along Lost Lookout Trail provides an inspiring view of Ausable Lake and a particularly interesting view of Rainbow Falls, which marks the end of this leg of the trip.

To reach Lost Lookout Trail, climb up the log ladder on the other side of Beaver Meadow Falls. As you climb alongside Beaver Meadow Falls, you can see its entirety. The trail, marked in blue, leads to Gothics and Armstrong mountains and climbs fairly steeply. You quickly reach the Lost Lookout fork on your left, which is marked in red disks and is 0.2 miles from Beaver Meadow Falls, 3.5 miles from the start. The trail climbs steadily through the beech-and-maple forest for another 0.3 miles, where you reach the first of two lookouts. You can see Ausable Lake, Indian Head, and Fish Hawk Cliffs nearby, as well as Bear Den, Dial, and Nippletop mountains, among other peaks visible to the south. The second lookout is nearby and offers the same views after traversing a short but steep descent. The trail continues southwest and descends for the next 0.8 miles. You will begin to hear the deep roar of the falls and glimpse the 150-foot waterfall. Extremely sheer drop-offs are to the side of the trail, so do not attempt to climb down to get to the falls from here. A separate trail farther ahead brings you to the base of Rainbow Falls. The trail winds down steeply for the next 0.3 miles, after which you reach the intersection with West River Trail. The trail marked in yellow quickly leads to a dam that marks the end of Ausable Lake and the head of the East Branch of Ausable River. After crossing Cascade Brook, you reach a long log-and-plank bridge that crosses the river below this dam and leads to East River Trail, as well as Indian Head and Fish Hawk Cliffs on the left. A trail to the right leads to Sawteeth and Gothics mountains, as well as Rainbow Falls. You will return to this point, 4.9 miles from the start, so that you can head back along East River Trail.

Before returning, take the blue-marked trail to the right to see these spectacular falls, less than 0.3 miles away. Shortly after

Rainbow Falls seen from Lost Lookout Trail

beginning along the blue trail, you reach a fork with a yellow-marked trail that indicates Sawteeth Mountain (via the scenic route) on the left and Gothics Mountain, Sawteeth Mountain (presumably along a hideous stretch of trail), and Rainbow Falls off to the right on the blue trail. A few hundred feet later, the trail to Gothics and the others, marked in blue, diverges to the left, while the path to the falls continues to your right but is now marked sporadically in red. You will pass several pipes, both plastic and steel, as you weave your way through boulders to the base of the sheer cliffs that form the falls. A sheer rock wall forms on your left as you work your way up alongside Cascade Brook to the base of Rainbow Falls. The canyon formed by the sheer rock walls amplifies the thundering of the falls as the water drops 150 feet. Mist sprayed on the opposing wall provides a haven for moss, while the water has scoured clean the rock wall on the waterfall side. The contrast of verdant green and jet black on the opposing walls is a unique scene that invites lingering. Head back to the dam to reach East River Trail as well as the spectacular views from Indian Head and Fish Hawk Cliffs.

DIRECTIONS: Coming from the south along NY 73, look for Ausable Club Road on your left just after descending a steep hill, 5.9 miles north of the intersection of US 9 and NY 73 in New Russia. Coming from the north, this end of Ausable Club Road is on your right, 3 miles south of the High Peaks sign in Keene Valley. This end of Ausable Club Road (the road intersects NY 73 a second time farther north) is directly across from the Giant Mountain parking area described on page 256. The parking area is almost immediately on your left after you turn onto Ausable Club Road.

GPS Parking Area Coordinates	35 Ausable River: West River Trail
UTM Zone (WGS 84):	18T
Easting:	0598532.0
Northing:	4889246.1
Latitude:	N 44° 08' 59.19"
Longitude:	W 73° 46' 4.53"

GPS Trailhead Coordinates	35 Ausable River: West River Trail
UTM Zone (WGS 84):	18T
Easting:	0597447.7
Northing:	4889240.5
Latitude:	N 44° 08' 59.53"
Longitude:	W 73° 46' 53.33"

36 Ausable River: *East River Trail*

SCENERY: ☆ ☆ ☆ ☆	DISTANCE: *4.3 miles one way; 1.6-mile side trip*
TRAIL CONDITION: ☆ ☆ ☆ ☆ ☆	HIKING TIME: *3–4 hours one way*
CHILDREN: ☆ ☆ ☆	OUTSTANDING FEATURES: *Scenic views,*
DIFFICULTY: ☆ ☆ ☆	*dramatic cliffs, spectacular waterfall, riverside stroll*
SOLITUDE: ☆ ☆ ☆ ☆	

The East River Trail is the return leg of a loop along the East Branch of Ausable River. Fewer waterfalls are along this section, but it does include a side trip to Indian Head and Fish Hawk Cliffs, which have impressive views and dramatic scenery of their own. Be advised that this hike lies on private property (public access has been granted), so certain restrictions apply (see West River Trail, page 236, for details on the restrictions).

🏃 You can hike the east section of Ausable River on its own, but I found it to be an excellent return trip for West River Trail. A side trip to Indian Head and Fish Hawk Cliffs reveals amazing views and is well worth the extra 1.6 miles. Directions back to the parking area along NY 73 and for the side trip are given from the end of West River Trail. From the intersection of West River Trail with the trail that leads to Sawteeth and Gothics mountains and Rainbow Falls, proceed east across the long bridge. On the other side of Ausable River, you intersect East River Trail to your left and a path to your right that heads uphill to Lake Road, as well as the trail to Indian Head and Fish Hawk Cliffs. Mileage given is from this point and not from the total loop or as the summation of the side trip to the cliffs.

INDIAN HEAD AND FISH HAWK CLIFFS

As you head uphill, you pass a maintenance building on your left and, shortly after, reach Lake Road. The road continues downhill to your right to where Adirondack Mountain Reserve (AMR) members have access to Ausable Lake. Hikers are prohibited from entering

Nubble

Roaring Brook

Putnam Brook

Roaring Brook Trail

73

Westen Trail

Round Mountain

Round Pond Trail

N. Fork Bouquet River

DIX MOUNTAIN WILDERNESS

Dix Trail

Noonmark Mountain

Senson Trail

Dix Trail

To Keene

73

P

Ausable Club Rd.

E. Branch Ausable River

CR 8A

AMR gate

Leach Trail

ADIRONDACK STATE PARK

Bear Den Mountain

Snow Mountain Trail

Ladies Mile Trail

Cathedral Rocks

Lake Rd.

Wedge Brook Cascades

Artists Falls

Deer Brook

W. A. White Trail

Cathedral Rocks and Bear Run Trail

waterfall lookout

Gill Brook

Gill Brook Trail

Indian Head Trail

Hedgehog Mountain

Wedge Brook Trail

Beaver Meadows Falls

maintenance building

Indian Head

Indian Head Lookout

HIGH PEAKS WILDERNESS

Lower Wolfjaw Mountain

W. A. White Trail

West River Trail

Lower Wolf Trail

ADR Range Trail

Upper Wolfjaw Mountain

Beaver Meadows Trail

Lost Lookout Trail

Rainbow Falls

Lower Ausable Lake

Armstrong Mountain

A. E. Weld Trail

trail fork to Gothics

trail fork to Sawteeth

Scenic Trail

this area, so be mindful and keep on the designated trails. Head a short distance east along the road, and look for the trailhead on your right. The trail is marked with yellow disks, and you quickly reach what appears to be a fork in the trail. However, the trail on the right leads to an AMR boathouse and is private, so keep to the left. The trail has several switchbacks that make the ascent a little more enjoyable than the typical rocky and straight scrambles to the top found on most Adirondacks trails. However, the trail is still considered steep, and several ladders have been built where short vertical sections over mossy and slick ledges would otherwise be difficult.

Approximately 0.3 miles in, you reach a fork in the trail and a sign indicating "Gothics Window—117 feet" to your right. The "window" is a slightly obscured view through the trees to the exposed portions of the Gothics. Saplings threaten to engulf the view and, though interesting, more-impressive views are farther along the trail. The side trip doesn't take long, though, so you will probably find it worth the diversion.

You reach the first of the ladders shortly after this fork, and the zigzags become tight and more frequent. After climbing several ladders and switchbacks, the trail levels off briefly under the base of a mossy cliff that adds a neat feature along the trail. Views of the Gothics are more prominent now, and the trail, though steep, has fewer turns in it.

At 0.8 miles, you reach the crest of the ridge and a four-way intersection. To the left is Gill Brook Trail, straight ahead and down leads to Fish Hawk Cliffs, and to the right is the trail to Indian Head. The trail is now encompassed by thick evergreens, and you briefly traverse the spine of this ridge before coming out on the exposed portions of the cliff that make up Indian Head. Spectacular views open up all around you, and you will quickly snap a dozen pictures. Rugged peaks with sheer cliffs fill the panorama to the north and west, but the most stunning views are of Lower Ausable Lake cradled between Colvin and Sawteeth mountains. Continue along the exposed portion of bedrock along worn footpaths to a second lower tier for a slightly different vantage point of the same spectacular view.

To reach Fish Hawk Cliffs, go back to the four-way intersection and head down the trail, which is now on your right. The descent is steep and takes you down 160 feet into a col near a pool called Wizard's Washbowl. Shortly ahead, 0.3 miles from the four-way intersection, you reach the cliffs, from which you have the unique perspective of looking back upon Indian Head. To return, go back to the four-way intersection and straight down to Lake Road and then East River Trail.

EAST RIVER TRAIL

East River Trail has fewer waterfalls than the west one but has its own unique character and elements that make it an excellent return trip. The trail meanders along the river briefly and then diverges east into the surrounding woods. Approximately 0.3 miles from the bridge, you navigate through a jumble of boulders that lie at the base of a cliff on your right. Shortly after, you pass Bullock Dam on your left. Following the dam, the river levels off and flows through a grassy meadow. On the opposite shore, you see exposed cliffs and many views of the mountains to the west.

Just shy of a mile, you reach a fork in the trail; Beaver Meadow and Gothics are to your left over a bridge and marked in blue, while the East River Trail and road, marked in red, continue straight ahead. Almost immediately after this intersection, you reach yet another fork, with East River Trail continuing straight ahead and the road to your right.

The trail delves into tall and thick hemlocks, and you soon reach a beautiful waterfall along the river. You might remember seeing this more than 20-foot-high waterfall and its constricted flume from the opposite shore. However, on this shore, there are far better points to view the falls and its washed-out spillway. You are now high above the river canyon, and this is one of the last points from which to view the river. Farther on, you hear the rumble of the turbulent waters but will only have glimpses of the river from afar, as the trail winds its way back down to the gatehouse.

The trail becomes steep in a few sections but levels off about 2.5 miles from the start. Gill Brook joins you on your right, and shortly after this, you will cross the brook over a bridge built from two sturdy beams. Soon after the bridge, you rejoin Ausable River as it flows northeast, and the trail follows the river 0.3 miles. At 3.1 miles, you reach another fork. Straight ahead is a bridge to West River Trail, while to your right is East River Trail and the path back to the road. In 0.1 mile, you will come in sight of the road. Follow it back to the gatehouse to sign out and then back to the parking area by NY 73, completing a trip of 4.3 miles from the bridge at Ausable Lake, 10 miles to complete the loop, and a total of 11.6 miles, including the side trip.

DIRECTIONS: The trail begins at the end of West River Trail, so the parking area is the same.

Coming from the south along NY 73, look for Ausable Club Road on your left just after descending a steep hill, 5.9 miles north of the intersection of US 9 and NY 73 in New Russia. Coming from the north, this end of Ausable Club Road is on your right, 3 miles south of the High Peaks sign in Keene Valley. This end of Ausable Club Road (the road intersects NY 73 a second time farther north) is directly across from the Giant Mountain parking area described on page 256. The parking area is almost immediately on your left after you turn onto Ausable Club Road.

GPS Parking Area Coordinates	36 Ausable River: East River Trail
UTM Zone (WGS 84):	18T
Easting:	0598532.0
Northing:	4889246.1
Latitude:	N 44° 08' 59.19"
Longitude:	W 73° 46' 4.53"
GPS Trailhead Coordinates	36 Ausable River: East River Trail
UTM Zone (WGS 84):	18T
Easting:	0597447.7
Northing:	4889240.5
Latitude:	N 44° 08' 59.53"
Longitude:	W 73° 46' 53.33"

37 Giant's Nubble

SCENERY: 🐾 🐾 🐾 🐾 🐾	DISTANCE: *4.4 miles*
TRAIL CONDITION: 🐾 🐾 🐾 🐾	HIKING TIME: *3–4 hours*
CHILDREN: 🐾 🐾	OUTSTANDING FEATURES: *Spectacular*
DIFFICULTY: 🐾 🐾 🐾 🐾	*waterfall, primitive campsites, outstanding views*
SOLITUDE: 🐾 🐾 🐾	

This excellent trip combines a tall waterfall, scenic outlook, and picturesque pond within a very short distance. Don't let the distance or description fool you though; the rugged trail provides you with plenty of climbing, along with the majestic scenery that is associated with the High Peaks region.

🐾🐾 The asphalt parking area is tucked away on your right as you come down a steep hill along NY 73, so watch the odometer and be ready to make a sharp right. The parking area can easily accommodate a dozen cars, but if it's full, there is room on the shoulder of NY 73 or across the road in the Ausable River parking area (see its description on page 243).

The register and trailhead are at the eastern end of the lot. The trail is broad and flat, and you can just barely glimpse Roaring Brook through hardwoods off to the right. During the peak of summer, the brook runs dry and indicates that the falls ahead may not be as majestic as during rainy conditions or during the winter melt. About 0.1 mile in, you reach a fork in the trail. To the right is the trail to the base of Roaring Brook Falls, while to the left, the trail climbs to the top of the falls, Giant's Nubble, Giant's Washbowl, and Giant Mountain.

THE BASE OF ROARING BROOK FALLS

Continue to the right past the sheer rock wall on your left until you reach Roaring Brook. Straight across the brook are four designated campsites. These sprawling sites lie under a thick canopy of tall

37 **Giant's Nubble**

N

0   0.15   0.3
mile

Roaring Brook

Giant's Nubble

rock outcropping

Giant's Washbow

To Elizabethtown

73

Chapel Pond

ADIRONDACK STATE PARK

GIANT MOUNTAIN WILDERNESS

73

Weston Trail

Dix Trail

Semson Trail

Roaring Brook Falls

Roaring Brook

Putnam Brook

Ausable Rd.

To Keene

73

P

hemlocks, and each has a large stone fire pit. They are shielded from view of the falls by a steep hill to the north but are fairly close to another stream, the outflow of Chapel Pond. The sound of the stream and the thundering of the falls will likely drown out the sound of the road, which is still close by, though the occasional loud vehicle might disturb the tranquil setting. To reach the falls, you have to scramble up the rocky brook a very short distance. The falls, the entirety of which can be seen from the road, are nearly 325 feet high, depending on where you measure the start. They cascade in three tiers, with only the lowest section visible at the base.

GIANT'S NUBBLE, GIANT'S WASHBOWL, AND GIANT MOUNTAIN

The trail climbs steadily from the fork and passes a tiny lookout shortly after you begin the ascent. After the first section of climbing, the trail levels off briefly and then climbs gently again as it winds briefly southward around the contours of the hillside. As the trail swings eastward again, views across the valley begin to sprawl out before you. Approximately 0.5 miles in, you reach a fork in the trail;

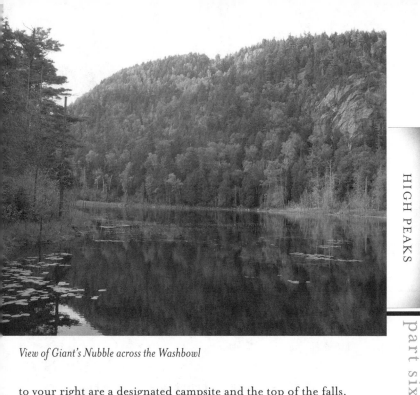

View of Giant's Nubble across the Washbowl

to your right are a designated campsite and the top of the falls, while straight ahead are Giant's Nubble, Giant's Washbowl, and the summit. The campsite, situated to the left of the falls path, is spacious, and there are plenty of spots to set up camp under the maple and ash canopy. To reach the top of the falls, follow any of the footpaths to Roaring Brook, and then rock-hop downstream. From the top of the falls, very little of the waterfall is visible because the drop is so precipitous and the water flows through a deep cleft in the bedrock. However, there are spectacular views out to the western horizon. The rocks at the top of the falls have been worn smooth by innumerable visitors and slope gradually toward a sheer drop-off, so use extra caution, especially during wet conditions.

Exposed bedrock at the Nubble

The main trail, marked by red disks, continues to head east and climbs steadily for the next 0.5 miles, where you reach another fork. To the left are two more designated campsites, both of which are situated under a heavy canopy of hemlocks and offer lots of room to set up. Shortly after this intersection, you wind around a large boulder and then turn quickly south as you rock-hop across Roaring Brook. On the opposite bank, you reach yet another fork. The trail to your left leads to Giant Mountain summit, 2.5 miles, while the nubble and washbowl are off to your right. Trail signs indicate that the nubble and washbowl are both 0.9 miles away, but the actual mileage is roughly 0.3 miles less. A tenth of a mile ahead, you reach the fork where the trails to the nubble and washbowl diverge from each other. This is also the terminus of the loop around both features and a return point back to NY 73. A trail sign indicates that the nubble is still 0.9 miles ahead while the washbowl is 0.8 miles ahead on the right. You can hike the loop in either direction, though I recommend hiking the nubble first, as there are some truly excellent views of the washbowl as you descend.

The trail up to the nubble, now marked with yellow trail disks, is a bit rougher than sections previously covered but no more than the usual Adirondack trail. Looming off to your left is the southern exposed face of Giant Mountain, which can be glimpsed occasionally through the surrounding fir trees. Many portions of the trail traverse moss-covered bedrock, and you pass by a square ledge of this oddly lush rock on your right shortly before you reach the fork in the trail, at 1.6 miles, that leads to the nubble. Veering right at the fork, you quickly reach the southeastern tip of the nubble, and a vast panorama of the eastern High Peaks opens up before you. Footpaths weave in and out of the exposed lichen-covered bedrock and wind-stunted fir trees as you make your way to the northern tip of the nubble. The lookout reveals a panorama of the northern High Peaks, as well as a beautiful vista of Giant Mountain off to the east. If the drive into the region did not give you an appreciation of the ruggedness of this area, then the views from atop the nubble certainly will.

The descent to the washbowl, initially marked with yellow disks, can be quite steep but has numerous lookouts as well. Less than 0.3 miles from the nubble is a truly excellent lookout that practically sits directly above the washbowl. The almost jet-black basin is nestled in a long depression between the base of the nubble, and a ridgeline before the slope of the mountain precipitously drops more than 800 feet to the valley floor in less than a third of a mile. From this vantage point, the pond seems to simply hang in the air. The trail weaves its way down through evergreens to the intersection with Giant's Ridge Trail at 2.1 miles. A green-and-white trail sign marks the intersection and indicates that the washbowl is a mere 0.3 miles farther on your right. The trail is heavily trodden but well maintained, and you quickly pass another designated campsite on your left, shortly before reaching the southeastern tip of the washbowl. A path along the eastern shore of the pond leads to another designated campsite that sits close to the water's edge, but the main trail winds to your left. You quickly pass the last intersection along this loop, where trail signs indicate that the Chapel Pond parking area along NY 73 is 0.7 miles ahead on your left, marked in blue markers, while the trail back to Roaring Brook Falls continues to your right, with red markers. The rocky nubble looms over the washbowl and provides some dramatic scenery as you hike along the western ridge that contains the pond. The brief shoreline hike northward is basically flat and rocky, with numerous rocks jutting out on the pond, all of which provide excellent points to view the pond and nubble. After leaving the washbowl's shore, you climb briefly along the base of the nubble and then begin your descent back to the beginning of the nubble and washbowl loop.

DIRECTIONS: Coming from the south along NY 73, look for the parking area on your right, just after descending a steep hill, 5.9 miles north of the intersection of US 9 and NY 73 in New Russia. Coming from the north, the parking area is on your left, 3 miles south of the High Peaks sign in Keene Valley. The parking area is directly across from the southern intersection of Ausable Road and NY 73.

GPS Trailhead Coordinates	37 Giant's Nubble
UTM Zone (WGS 84):	18T
Easting:	0598595.1
Northing:	4889319.9
Latitude:	N 44° 09' 1.55"
Longitude:	W 73° 46' 1.64"

38 Indian Pass

SCENERY: ✿ ✿ ✿ ✿ ✿	DISTANCE: *8.8 miles*
TRAIL CONDITION: ✿ ✿ ✿ ✿	HIKING TIME: *5–6 hours*
CHILDREN: ✿ ✿ ✿	OUTSTANDING FEATURES: *Maze of boulders,*
DIFFICULTY: ✿	*sheer cliffs, panoramic views*
SOLITUDE: ✿ ✿ ✿	

The trail leading to Indian Pass is, in its own right, an enjoyable excursion, and you can't help but feel the remoteness of the High Peaks Wilderness that surrounds you. The first three quarters of the trail is, however, not that different than many deep-woods hikes. It's the last 0.8 miles that really sets this trail apart and makes it a must-have adventure. After navigating your way through a maze of enormous boulders, you soon reach Summit Rock, and the spectacle of Wallface Mountain is truly impressive.

🚶 The Upper Works parking area for Indian Pass is quite large and easily accommodates dozens of vehicles. Indeed, it is one of the major access points for the High Peaks Wilderness and all the adventure that the area encompasses. The trail, marked with yellow disks, begins to the right of the trail register in the northeast corner of the lot. The trail starts along a gravelly road within the boundaries of the Tahawus Preserve, a vast area of wilderness that was acquired by the Open Space Institute in 2003, with major sections now jointly managed by the institute and the DEC. After 0.3 miles, you reach a wooden bridge sturdy enough for vehicles to cross. Congratulations! You have just crossed the Hudson River at its headwater. Just after the bridge, the road forks, with the trail continuing on the right. At a little more than 0.3 miles, you enter a meadow with a fork in the trail. The trail to the left leads to Duck Hole and Indian Pass, marked with yellow disks, while the trail to the right, marked with red disks, is Calamity Brook Trail and Mt. Marcy via Lake Colden. Calamity Brook Trail is also the return trip if you decide to take an extended

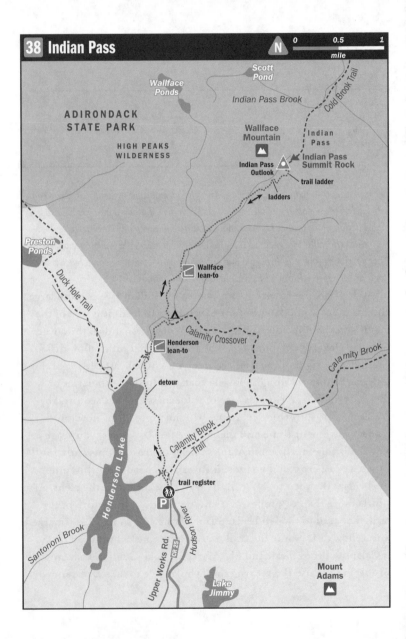

N

0   0.5   1

mile

Scott Pond

Wallface Ponds

Indian Pass Brook

Cold Brook Trail

ADIRONDACK STATE PARK

HIGH PEAKS WILDERNESS

Wallface Mountain

Indian Pass

Indian Pass Outlook

Indian Pass Summit Rock

trail ladder

ladders

Preston Ponds

Duck Hole Trail

Wallface lean-to

Calamity Crossover

Calamity Brook

Henderson lean-to

detour

Calamity Brook Trail

Henderson Lake

trail register

Santononi Brook

P

Upper Works Rd.

CR 25

Hudson River

Lake Jimmy

Mount Adams

trip, day or overnight, by crossing over the MacIntyre Mountains via Cold Brook Pass.

Continue along the left trail, which is a mostly open road with occasional views of Lake Henderson on your left. The road has many muddy areas, and regrowth encroaches on the road in several places. At 1.1 miles, you encounter what appears to be a fork in the trail but is actually a route around a mucky area. Choose the right path to avoid the worst of the mud. Just after this rerouting, you come close to Lake Henderson again, but thick hemlocks obscure most of the view.

Indian Pass Brook now flows off to your left, and at 1.5 miles, you reach another fork in the trail. At this point, you leave the broad road and stick to the foot trails. To the left is a log-and-plank bridge, and signs indicate that the Duck Hole lean-to is 5.3 miles and Coreys, 23.3 miles. Similarly, the sign indicates Henderson lean-to is 0.2 miles, Indian Pass is 2.7 miles, and the Adirondak Loj is 10.4 miles straight ahead. (The mileage to the Loj must include a detour because a straight path along the entire Indian Pass Trail brings you to the Loj in 10.4 miles, and you have already hiked 1.5 miles.)

Continue straight along mostly flat terrain, now marked with red disks. In 1.7 miles, you pass the Henderson lean-to on your left. On a Saturday morning, this lean-to is usually filled with hikers, who start late on Friday and want to get moving early. After reaching a meadow, Indian Pass Brook is again within sight, and you quickly reach the last fork of this trip, 2.1 miles. Signs indicate that to the left, Wallface lean-to is 0.6 miles, Indian Pass is 2.3 miles, and the Adirondak Loj is 6 miles. (Once again, the mileage to the Loj seems to be mistaken, but the others are correct.) The trail straight ahead, marked in blue, is the Calamity Brook Crossover trail, with Calamity Brook, 2.1 miles, and Lake Colden, 6 miles.

After taking the left trail, marked in red, you quickly reach a bridge over Indian Pass Brook. The recently constructed bridge has round rails and posts, as well as a large rock-filled crib on the opposite shore. Shortly after reaching the opposing shore, you pass a minor fork in the trail and a yellow disk indicating a designated campsite to your right. Nestled among dense evergreen saplings, the site is close to the confluence of two streams. The site has a sheltered feel and is filled with the soft babbling sounds of the water nearby.

Indian Pass Brook now flows on your right, and though it is nearby, you don't really see the brook until you approach the Wallface lean-to, 2.7 miles. The trail passes within feet of the brook, and the lean-to is just to the left of the trail. This is perhaps an ideal spot to enjoy the brook, but if you plan to stay in the lean-to, then expect traffic. The trail is mostly flat, and you cross many seasonal feeder streams as you work your way northeast to the intersection of a seasonal stream and Indian Pass Brook. You cross and recross the stream in what is a muddy little delta extending about 0.1 mile. Once through this mire, Indian Pass Brook continues to flow on your right. The grade steadily increases, and soon a sheer rock wall begins to rise on your right. At 3.8 miles, a jumble of enormous boulders on the eastern shore invites exploration. This is fortunate, as the trail crosses over Indian Pass Brook at this point, but the markings for the crossing

Wallface lean-to beside the trail

are not that clear, and the exact crossover point is easily missed.

On the other shore, the trail becomes more rugged and climbs steeply in sections. The moss-covered giant boulders you are climbing through form myriad crevices, caves, and clefts that make for some interesting scenery and excellent exploration. As you climb, and after passing a 40-foot-high boulder on your right, you will begin to glimpse through the canopy to your left the sheer rock walls of Wallface Mountain. The scene is impressive and promises a dramatic vista ahead at Indian Pass Outlook. At 4.1 miles, you reach a series of short ladders that assist you up this steep section. The trail swings south briefly, then heads north again to the base of a much taller ladder at 4.3 miles. Once you are atop this ladder, it is a very short way to the fork that leads to the outlook on your left. A short ladder leads you a few dozen feet off the main trail to the Indian Pass Summit Rock outlook. From this rocky outcrop, you have an amazing view of the sheer cliffs of Wallface Mountain, as well as an expansive view down the valley to the south. Return the way you came for a total trip of 8.8 miles.

DIRECTIONS: County Road 25, the access road to the Upper Works/Tahawus parking area, can be reached 18 miles west of I-87 N, Exit 29, via CR 2-B/Boreas Road; 5 miles east of the town hall in Newcomb; or 7.3 miles north of Aiden Lair, along NY 28 N. CR 2-B/Boreas Road intersects CR 25 1.6 miles east of the intersection of CR 25 and NY 28 N. Continue north on CR 25 past the entrance to the Tahawus club, 0.4 miles, over the railroad tracks and a bridge over the Hudson River, 0.6 miles. At 6.3 miles, continue straight along CR 25-A (CR 25 continues east along a bridge over the Hudson). Continue north on CR 25-A past an old furnace on your right, 8.8 miles, and a parking area on your right, 9.3 miles, to the end of the road and the Upper Works parking area, 9.9 miles from the intersection of CR 25 and CR 2-B/Boreas Road.

GPS Trailhead Coordinates	38 Indian Pass
UTM Zone (WGS 84):	18T
Easting:	0575520.9
Northing:	4881969.2
Latitude:	N 44° 05' 20.24"
Longitude:	W 74° 03' 23.97"

39 Little and Big Crow Mountains

SCENERY: ✿ ✿ ✿ ✿ ✿	SOLITUDE: ✿ ✿ ✿
TRAIL CONDITION: ✿ ✿ ✿ ✿	DISTANCE: *3.3 miles*
CHILDREN: ✿ ✿ ✿	HIKING TIME: *2–3 hours*
DIFFICULTY: ✿ ✿ ✿	OUTSTANDING FEATURES: *Spectacular vistas*

This short trip is an excellent introductory hike for people who want to familiarize themselves with the beautiful vistas of the High Peaks, without spending a whole day. Both experts and novices will appreciate the wealth of views atop the many ledges you encounter as you weave your way to the summit.

🚶🚶 To make the trail into a loop, you will have to walk 1.4 miles along O'Toole Road and Hurricane Road. You can hike the road section either at the end or at the beginning of the hike, but I recommend hiking the trail clockwise and including the roadside portion at the beginning. The counterclockwise direction includes a steeper ascent to Big Crow and requires you to end your hike walking uphill along the road rather than ending the trail with a descent and flat stroll through the woods. The trail register is located a few hundred yards northwest of the parking area. To reach the western trailhead, walk down O'Toole Road and turn right onto Hurricane Road, 1.1 miles. Continue down Hurricane Road 0.2 miles, and look for a small orange ADK marker affixed to a wooden sign that points to the trail. This sign is difficult to see while driving but evident while on foot. The trail starts at a couple of log steps and winds around the left side of a private residence. This section of the trail is on private property, so be careful to stay on the marked portion of the trail.

Red trail disks mark the way, and you quickly begin to climb through a stand of small saplings. Roughly a half mile into the trail, 1.8 miles from the start, expansive views to the south and west begin

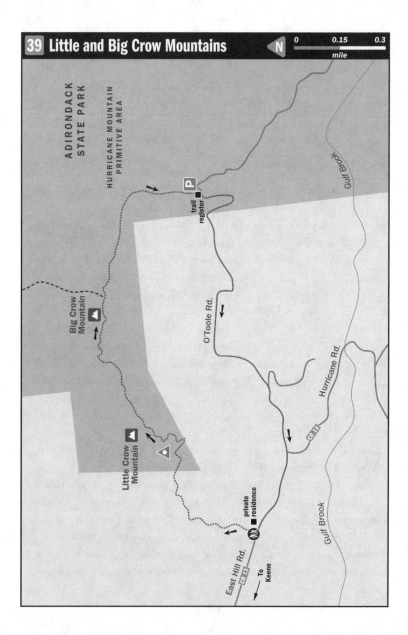

39 Little and Big Crow Mountains

N

0   0.15   0.3
mile

ADIRONDACK STATE PARK

HURRICANE MOUNTAIN PRIMITIVE AREA

Big Crow Mountain

Little Crow Mountain

Gulf Brook

O'Toole Rd.

Hurricane Rd.

CR 13

Gulf Brook

trail register

P

private residence

East Hill Rd.

CR 13

To Keene

to open up behind you. Exposed portions of bedrock begin to jut out, both making the terrain more rugged and forming natural steps as you climb. You will see yellow paint blazes on trees that may seem to guide you along the trail, but these are actually the boundary between private property and the DEC-designated primitive area.

A primitive area is a DEC land-use designation that is essentially the same as a wilderness area, in that recreation is limited to passive activities, such as hiking, camping, birding, angling, and hunting, that meet the leave-no-trace standards. Additional restrictions regarding the types of structures that are allowed differentiate a primitive area from a wilderness area. Perhaps the main difference is that wilderness areas must be a minimum of 5,000 contiguous acres, while primitive areas have no size requirement.

The exposed ledges along the trail all offer excellent views, but a particularly spectacular vista is available just past where you enter the public lands, 2 miles from the start. Take advantage of these lookouts, as the summit of Little Crow does not offer any views. Red disks and rock cairns help you navigate as you weave your way over exposed portions of bedrock and through windswept conifers. At 2.3 miles, the peak of Little Crow Mountain, 2,450 feet, is off to the left of the main trail. The bald top of Little Crow is quite exposed, but it is also a broad peak; consequently, the encircling evergreens limit views typical of a bald summit.

To reach Big Crow, continue west along the exposed bedrock, and then quickly descend the short pass between the two peaks. Big Crow appears more rugged as you approach, but the climb to Little Crow is actually the tougher of the two. The oak saplings that fill the pass are a pleasant diversion from the encompassing evergreens that shroud the mountaintops. Indeed, as you climb Big Crow, the conifers become so dense and so closely flank the trail that only the path ahead is visible. However, the dense foliage is brief, and a view to the north soon rewards your efforts. Whiteface Mountain, with its numerous ski slopes, is particularly prominent as you look northward. The trail turns southward, and an excellent lookout to the south and west quickly reveals the path you have taken. After a brief scramble up the exposed bedrock, you reach the beginning of the exposed spine that runs along the short ridge. A sweeping panorama of tall peaks extends from due east southward to due west as you traverse the ridge. The highest point on the trip, 2,800 feet, is 2.8 miles and is simply atop a boulder where a sign reminds visitors that no camping or fires are allowed at the peak. Continue east along the ridge to where the descent down the open face is rather steep. After approximately a quarter mile, the steep section is past, and the rest of the hike through the spruce forest feels very sheltered compared with the exposed peaks. At 3.2 miles, you cross a small brook, after which the trail is mostly level, and you quickly reach the trail register and return to the parking area approximately a quarter mile ahead.

DIRECTIONS: From NY 73 in Keene, head west on County Road 13/ Hurricane Road (1.7 miles north of the southern intersection of NY 73 and NY 9 N, and 0.2 miles south of the northern intersection of NY 73 and NY 9 N). Continue on CR 13/Hurricane Road 2.3 miles, and then turn left onto O'Toole Road. Follow O'Toole Road 1.1 miles to the parking area at the end.

GPS Parking Area Coordinates	39 Little and Big Crow Mountains
UTM Zone (WGS 84):	18T
Easting:	0601093.3
Northing:	4901709.3
Latitude:	N 44° 15' 41.78"
Longitude:	W 73° 44' 0.61"

GPS Trailhead Coordinates	Trailhead along Hurricane Road
UTM Zone (WGS 84):	18T
Easting:	0599821.5
Northing:	4901866.1
Latitude:	N 44° 15' 47.49"
Longitude:	W 73° 44' 57.85"

40 Pitchoff Mountain

SCENERY: ✿ ✿ ✿ ✿	DISTANCE: *4.6 miles*
TRAIL CONDITION: ✿ ✿ ✿ ✿	HIKING TIME: *5–6 hours*
CHILDREN: ✿ ✿ ✿	OUTSTANDING FEATURES: *Panoramic views,*
DIFFICULTY: ✿ ✿ ✿ ✿	*open ledges*
SOLITUDE: ✿ ✿ ✿	

This rocky ridge parallels NY 73 and provides excellent views of the High Peaks wilderness to the south. This is an end-to-end hike and easiest to manage with two cars—or park at one end and catch a ride to the other. There are several steep rock scrambles, so be prepared during wet and icy conditions.

🚶🚶 The two trailheads are 2.7 miles apart along NY 73. This is a major road with narrow shoulders, so it is advised that you either leave a vehicle at both ends or leave your car at one end and get a lift to the other. I would suggest getting a ride before your hike, rather than after, to avoid uncertainty and because the trail will likely take longer than is typical for the mileage. The west trailhead has more parking room, so it is best to leave your vehicle there and hike the trail from east to west. Directions below are given in that direction.

The east trailhead is little more than a worn path with a couple of steps that extend down to the road, but there are signs there, and it is distinct. The trail register is at the beginning of the trail, and even though you will sign in and out at different registers, it is still important to sign in and out. The trail, marked with red disks and yellow blazes for the whole trip, turns west almost immediately and parallels the road for roughly 0.3 miles under a canopy of birch and beech trees. The trail swings north, and you begin climbing amongst a jumble of cobbles and boulders alongside a rocky brook. The grade steadily increases and becomes a lot steeper 0.8 miles into the hike. At approximately 1 mile, you have almost reached the ridge that you

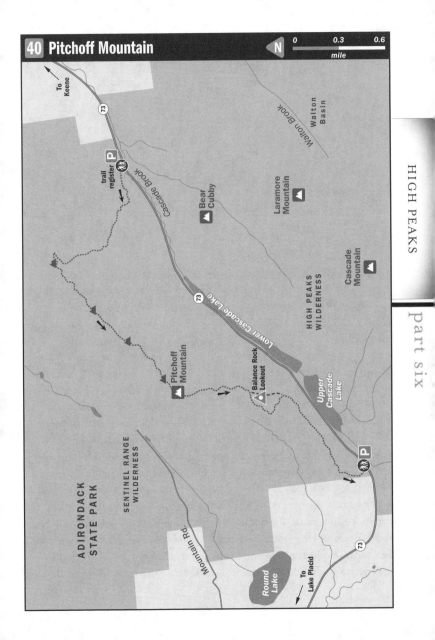

40 Pitchoff Mountain

N

0   0.3   0.6
mile

HIGH PEAKS

part six

To
Keene

73

P

trail
register

Cascade Brook

Bear
Cubby

Walton
Brook

Walton
Basin

Laramore
Mountain

Pitchoff Mountain

73

Lower Cascade Lake

Balance Rock
Lookout

HIGH PEAKS
WILDERNESS

Cascade
Mountain

Upper
Cascade
Lake

ADIRONDACK
STATE PARK

SENTINEL RANGE
WILDERNESS

Mountain Rd.

P

73

Round
Lake

To
Lake Placid

will traverse, and though many steep up-and-down sections are still ahead, the majority of the climbing is behind you. At 1.1 miles, you pass through a wet area between two 20- to 30-foot-high rocky outcrops that flank the trail. Once through this small pass, the trail turns left, and you scramble up to the top of one of these outcrops.

At 1.2 miles, you have reached the first of five minor peaks that comprise Pitchoff Mountain. Ridgelines with multiple peaks do not have separate mountain names if the prominence of a peak does not exceed 980 feet or 7 to 8 percent relative prominence above the highest saddle or col between the peaks. In ridges such as this one, with slight elevation differences between peaks and cols, it's clear why the distinction between mountains and peaks is useful. The trail weaves its way up and down many times before you reach the actual summit 1.5 miles ahead. The views to the south are exceptional, and many similar vantage points will accompany you as you traverse the spine. Yellow paint blazes mark the path along these bald peaks. If you are attempting this hike after a recent snowfall, finding your way can be time consuming. Snow falls as early as October and late into the spring in the High Peaks region. During the light snows of the

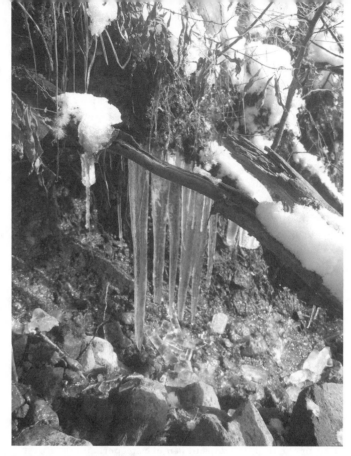

Icicles along the trail in early October

fall and thaws during spring, when the snow is not deep enough for snowshoes, you need crampons or their equivalent to cross the bald peaks. The cycles of thawing and freezing on the exposed rocky ledges and peaks produce sheets of ice that are treacherous without added traction. Pack accordingly, even though these conditions may not be evident down at the road.

The trail weaves up and down over boulders and zigzags through wind-stunted evergreens across the entire spine, and many times you will think that you have reached a peak, or traversed a pass between peaks, only to find yet another climb or pass before you. This is particularly true for the 0.5 miles between the first and second peaks. The second peak, 1.8 miles, offers a wide panoramic view to the south but does not offer the 360-degree views found at the first peak. The trail descends and climbs mostly along the ridgeline to the third peak at 2.1 miles, where there are also views to south.

Between the third and fourth summits, the trail meanders to the north side of the ridge, where the fir trees become thick, and then heads back to the south side. The fourth peak, 2.5 miles, is not the highest point of elevation but is the last peak with panoramic views. At 2.7 miles, you pass some balancing boulders that mark the fifth and final peak as well as the beginning of the steep descent from the ridgeline. Dense conifers shroud the trail for most of the descent, but occasional breaks in the trails and open ledges offer some views.

At 3.2 miles, you reach the only fork in the trail and a sign that indicates a "view" is off to the left. This lookout, approximately 0.1 mile along an unmarked path, is atop a sheer ledge with two balanced boulders that sit at its westernmost edge. Cascade Mountain and Upper and Lower Cascade lakes are the prominent features of the view, and the lookout is certainly worth the short side trip.

Back along the trail, the descent is much steeper, and the forest transitions back to hardwoods. The steep descent continues for about 0.5 miles, during which you pass under the sheer rock wall that makes up the lookout to your left. The trail turns westward, levels off, and parallels NY 73 and Upper Cascade Lake for the next 0.5 miles. At 4.3 miles, the trail swings south, and you descend for the next 0.3 miles until you reach the western trailhead and Upper Cascade Lake parking area.

Rocks and cobbles strewn across the trail's ascent to First Peak

DIRECTIONS: Parking is available at both the east and the west ends of Cascade Lake along NY 73. Parking is limited in both areas, and there is little room on the roadside. The parking areas are 2.7 miles apart along NY 73. The eastern parking area is 3.8 miles west of the northern intersection of NY 73 and NY 9 N in Keene. The western parking area is 5.5 miles east of the intersection of County Road 12 and NY 73. This intersection is near the Olympic Ski Jump in Lake Placid.

Snowfall in the small pass before First Peak

GPS Trailhead Coordinates	**40 Pitchoff Mountain/East**
UTM Zone (WGS 84):	18T
Easting:	0592151.8
Northing:	4899592.5
Latitude:	N 44° 14' 37.46"
Longitude:	W 73° 50' 45.13"
GPS Trailhead Coordinates	**40 Pitchoff Mountain/West**
UTM Zone (WGS 84):	18T
Easting:	0588902.8
Northing:	4896828.9
Latitude:	N 44° 13' 9.36"
Longitude:	W 73° 53' 13.28"

Appendix A: Managing Agencies

NEW YORK STATE DEPARTMENT OF ENVIRONMENTAL CONSERVATION

dec.ny.gov
625 Broadway
Albany, NY 12233-0001
(530) 622-5061
(518) 473-9518

NEW YORK STATE ADIRONDACK PARK AGENCY

apa.state.ny.us
P.O. Box 99
1133 NY 86
Ray Brook, NY 12977
(518) 891-4050

Appendix B: Gear Lists

DAY HIKE GEAR LIST
The Essentials
Backpack

Boots

Extra food

First-aid kit

Flashlight and extra batteries

Pocketknife or multitool

This book

Topographical map and compass

Water bottles

Water filter or purification tablets

Waterproof matches and/or lighter,
as well as a fire starter

Whistle

Additional
Change of clothes

Extra socks

Insect repellent

Personal medications

Poncho or raingear

UV sunblock and lip balm

Warm hat

Optional
Camera with extra batteries and
memory/film

Gaiters

Garbage bag for packing out trash

GPS unit

Repair kit

Small towel

Swimsuit

Survival kit

Toilet paper

Trowel or small shovel for
digging catholes

SUMMER BACKPACKING GEAR LIST
Backpack

Bear bag or canister

Cleaning supplies—biodegradable
detergent and container, sponge,
and scouring pad

Collapsible bucket or water bag

Collapsible pillow

Cooking pots and pans

Eating utensils—cup, bowl, plate,
knife, fork, and spoon

50 feet of rope and nylon cord

Food—including extra for
emergencies

Garbage bag for packing out trash

Shelter and conveyance

Sleeping bag and sleeping pad
or mattress

Stove and fuel

Tent and rain fly

Tent stakes

Water bottles

Water filter or purification tablets

Waterproof matches and/or lighter,
as well as a fire starter

Personal Items

Biodegradable hand soap

First-aid kit

Insect repellent

Small towel

Personal medications

Toilet paper

Toothbrush and toothpaste

Trowel or small shovel for
digging catholes

UV sunblock and lip balm

Gear

Camera with extra batteries and
memory/film

Camp light or candle

Flashlight and extra batteries

GPS unit

Pocketknife or multitool

Repair kit

Sewing kit

Stuff sacks

Survival kit

This book

Topographical map and compass

Whistle

Clothing

Boots

Camp shoes

Extra socks

Gaiters

Jacket or outerwear
(layer clothing)

Light shirt or T-shirt

Long pants

Poncho or raingear

Separate plastic bag for laundry

Shorts

Sock liners

Swimsuit

Warm hat

Warm shirt

Appendix C: Suggested Reading

Dunn, Russell. *Adirondack Waterfall Guide: New York's Cool Cascades.*
Hensonville, NY: Black Dome Press Corp., 2004.

Ketchledge, Edwin H. *Forests & Trees of the Adirondack High Peaks Region:
A Hiker's Guide.* Lake George, NY: Adirondack Mountain Club, 1996.

Van Diver, Bradford B. *Roadside Geology of New York.* Missoula, MT:
Mountain Press Publishing Company, 1985.

Wells, Catherine with Aaron Starmer and Timothy Starmer.
The Best in Tent Camping: New York State. Birmingham, AL: Menasha Ridge
Press, 2007.

Index

Since its founding in 1976, **American Hiking Society** has been the only national voice for hikers—dedicated to promoting and protecting America's hiking trails, their surrounding natural areas and the hiking experience. **American Hiking Society** works every day:

- Speaking for hikers in the halls of Congress and with federal land managers
- Building and maintaining hiking trails
- Educating and supporting hikers by providing information and resources
- Supporting hiking and trail organizations nationwide

Whether you're a casual hiker or a seasoned backpacker, become a member of **American Hiking Society** and join the national hiking community! You'll not only enjoy great members-only benefits but you will help ensure the hiking trails you love will remain protected and will be waiting for you the next time you lace up your boots and hit the trail.

We invite you to join us today!

1422 Fenwick Lane · Silver Spring, MD 20910 · (800) 972-8608
www.AmericanHiking.org · info@AmericanHiking.org

About the Author

TIM STARMER has always been an outdoor enthusiast and spent most of his
childhood seeking out remote and wild
areas whenever possible. During a brief
hiatus from Brown University during 1997, he drove across the United
States for six weeks, camping the entire
way. Along the way he explored many
of the West's national and state parks,
including Canyonlands, Yellowstone, Arches, and Bryce Canyon—he
even braved pitching a tent among the mosquito swarms in Badlands
National Park. At the trip's conclusion, he headed down to Australia,
where he backpacked for a few months exploring the eastern outback,
the Great Barrier Reef, and the caves of Tasmania, as well as traversing the Tasmanian World Heritage Area along the Overland Track.
Starmer owns and operates New Heritage Woodworking, a construc-
tion company that specializes in designing and building timber frames,
and he can still be found exploring the wilds whenever possible.